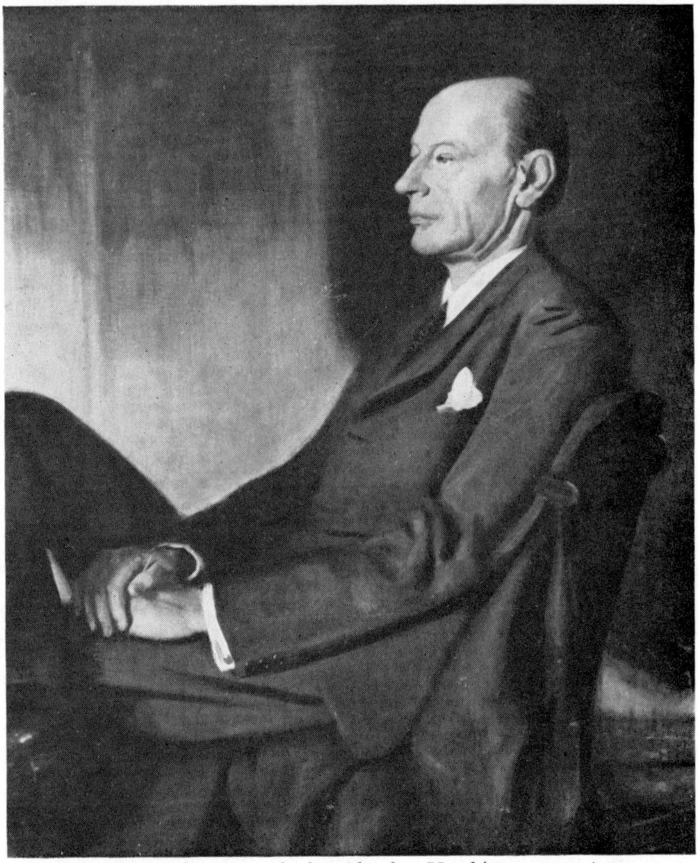

(From the portrait by Charles Hopkinson, 1940)

GEORGE RICHARDS MINOT

THE INQUISITIVE PHYSICIAN

THE INQUISITIVE PHYSICIAN

THE LIFE AND TIMES OF

George Richards Minot, A.B. M.D. D.Sc.

By

Francis M. Rackemann, A.B. M.D.

Seest thou a man diligent in his business?
He shall stand before kings.
PROVERBS 23:29

HARVARD UNIVERSITY PRESS
Cambridge, Massachusetts
1956

Distributed in Great Britain by

Geoffrey Cumberlege, Oxford University Press, London

Library of Congress Catalog Card Number: 56–6521

Printed in the United States of America

TO HIS WIFE

MARIAN WELD MINOT

Preface

George Richards Minot was a physician who discovered the liver treatment of pernicious anemia and received the Nobel Prize for his achievement. Every student of medicine knows this, but it is only a part — even though the glamorous part — of his life.

George Minot was inquisitive about almost everything in nature. His field was the blood: he cultivated it intensively to make wonderful crops, and at the same time he cleared the forest to make the field larger.

Right in the middle of his most active investigations, he developed diabetes, which in those days was serious, and then comes a very dramatic story. The discovery of insulin was made just in time to save his life, so that he in turn could make his own discovery of the liver treatment. Thanks to his infinite capacity for taking pains, as Thomas Carlyle has defined genius, pernicious anemia is pernicious no longer.

Since he became Professor of Medicine, about four hundred young doctors have been trained at the Thorndike Memorial Laboratory, chiefly under his guidance — and trained so well that over one hundred of them have been chosen to hold high academic positions in the medical schools of the world. If the success of former students is an index of the ability of the teacher, George R. Minot stands in the first rank.

His students, and their students in turn, inherit something of his understanding and love of his fellow men. They, too, are inquisitive physicians.

The span of George Minot's life was the period of extraordinary intellectual, technological, material, and social progress. When in 1912 and 1913 George and I were "House Pupils" at the Massachusetts General Hospital there were no "Residents" — no other "full-time" young men working in the hospital. Almost no clinical research was in progress. When now one sees the modern research institutes — whole buildings filled with laboratories containing apparatus and facilities of every kind — and sees the chemists, physicists, and biologists, as well as the physicians, who are working in them, the change which has come about in our lifetime — which we have seen with our own eyes — is remarkable. It is thrilling, and yet this is but another step in our progress.

See what Sir William Osler said at the dedication of the Phipps Clinic at Johns Hopkins in 1913: "To have lived through a revolution, to have seen a new birth of science, a new dispensation of health, reorganized medical schools, remodeled hospitals, a new outlook for humanity, is not given to every generation." Little did he know that the very next generation — ours — was to see an even greater change. We can only guess at what our sons will see.

George Minot and I were cousins. We grew up together. He and I went to school together, we were in college at the same time, and then were very close in medical school and hospital. When he went to Baltimore and I went to New York, for our special studies, our ways parted a little, but we were never out of touch. Our wives are devoted to each other, and our children are as intimate as we were. It is very pleasant to review what we did together in the early days and then to try to describe the development of my friend who became such a distinguished man.

His wife, Marian Weld Minot, played a large part in his remarkable life. She took care of his diabetes, supervising his food and his insulin. She reviewed his papers and criticized his addresses. George never traveled anywhere without her. She helped him to cultivate his irises; she guarded his library — its "atmosphere" as well as the books it contained. She kept a difficult household running smoothly. Guests were invited in appropriate numbers and in congenial, interesting combinations. Their three children grew up to be a great credit to them both.

To know George and Marian Minot so well has been a joy and a privilege, as well as a great stimulus. If in this book I have succeeded in sharing with others what I have learned from them, I will be pleased.

In writing this book, I have had help from many friends. Marian Minot has helped me greatly with ideas and suggestions. She gave me official permission to examine George's files. Dr. Elliott P. Joslin allowed me to study his record of George's case. Miss Anna S. Holt and her staff in the Harvard Medical School Library have helped me efficiently. A number of George's associates have written me letters or given me little items which illuminated George's character.

When the chapters began to take shape, Dr. William B. Castle read and corrected my technical passages. Dr. Francis T. Hunter, George's brother-in-law, studied the manuscript with care and made many excellent suggestions. It is unfortunate that he died before the book was ready. Dr. Cecil K. Drinker and Dr. James Howard Means seemed to be pleased with the first draft. When later Dr. Claude M. Fuess and Professor Howard Mumford Jones read a revised version, they were encouraging, even if they could see that still more changes must be made. Mrs. Charles P. Graves (George Minot's daughter Elizabeth), an experienced book reviewer, and Mrs. David E. Humez of the Harvard University Press helped me to make wise improvements. Mrs. Humez taught me much about the arrangement of a complex story.

To all of these I am very grateful, and I thank them. I thank also Mr. Joseph D. Elder, Science Editor of the Press, and other members of the staff for their kindly tolerance in raising and answering endless questions. I thank my secretary, Miss Eileen F. Dinan, for typing and retyping many pages. Finally, my wife has lived with the book for a longer time than either of us anticipated, and I appreciate her forbearance among her other virtues.

CONTENTS

THE INQUISITIVE PHYSICIAN

1

In the Beginning

On a Sunday afternoon in Massachusetts in May 1896, Dr. and Mrs. James Jackson Minot had just moved their three small sons — George, ten, Jimmy, four, and Henry, a baby of only three months — out from Boston to Milton for the summer. My mother and father let me, a boy of nine, drive over with them behind Molly in the green wagon to call on the Minots. In front of the Minot house there was a garden, with flowers near the driveway and vegetables farther back; George's father, my "Cousin Jim," had given George a small corner of one of the flower beds for his own. The little seedlings were coming up, and George was both pleased and proud. I knew nothing about plants, and when I stepped on one of the little shoots George didn't like it. Words were followed by blows, and in the course of the struggle we moved nearer the water barrel. Whether George put me into the water barrel, or whether I put him in, was a question that has been debated many times. One could hardly say that our friendship began in any very propitious manner, but it developed nevertheless. Obviously it began early.

Cousin Jim was a small man, quiet, reserved, and dignified, who took life seriously. He was stern and strict; at first I was afraid of him. He was not a strong healthy man and he worried about himself and about other things, too. He was alarmed by the water-barrel episode, fearing lest we boys catch cold because of our wet clothes.

George's mother, my "Cousin Bessie," was eight years younger than her husband. She was full of fun and frolic, and she laughed at us as she tried to soothe her husband. What a friendly lady she was! She was always kind to me, and that was one reason why I came to love her. She found it hard to worry about the water barrel, because the Minots had just come out of the hot city, and the country air in May seemed pleasant and healthy. My mother agreed with her.

In those days, the well-established, well-to-do families of Boston lived in town on the western slope of Beacon Hill or just below it in the Back Bay. The Back Bay is so called because it is land that was filled in after 1857 behind the mill dam that once extended from the foot of the Hill about two miles along the Charles River, up to Sewall's Point in the suburb of Brookline. The eastern, or town, half of this land was settled by the lawyers, the merchants, the builders, and the doctors, in a rectangular area about a mile long and about half a mile wide, where the streets were leisurely, straight, and wide, where the brick sidewalks were uneven, and where trees grew in front of the houses. Commonwealth Avenue, in the center of the area, was divided into east and west drives by the "middle row" with its four lines of elms shading the central walk.

Cousin Jim was a successful doctor, and his house and office at 188 Marlborough Street were in the middle of the Back Bay. It was a tall and narrow house, on the shady side of the street. It had windows only on the front and back, with bay windows on the second floor. In the middle of the house there was an open space extending up to a skylight five floors above. The stairs wound around this light-well. One entered through a long vestibule with several steps leading up to an inside front door. From a landing in the middle of the steps a small side door gave entrance to a tiny waiting room, and through that to the doctor's office.

There was no secretary, no typewriter, and no telephone, at least for some years. No appointments were made, except occasionally by letter or by personal call. The patients came during office hours — or at least I suppose they did, for the boys and I never saw them; we were out of the house for most of the day.

There were no electric lights when George and his brothers were growing up. The gas, with Welsbach burners, gave a good soft light. This gas was lit by an electric spark when two small wires from a battery were brought together by pulling a little chain. The device worked well most of the time. Cousin Jim used to explain to me: "Never blow out the gas; you shut it off when you turn this little valve to the right. Do you understand?"

The dining room was at the back of the street floor, over the basement kitchen. The front parlor on the second floor was cold

Victorian, and no one ever went into it, except on state occasions, but the library in back of it was quiet and homey. The dark-figured wall paper and the dark-green stain of the heavy woodwork would have made it a gloomy place if the open fire had not been burning slowly most of the time in its great bed of ashes. There were bookcases along the walls, with countless prints and photographs on top of the cases and on the tables in the center of the room. In spite of its somber color, the library was comfortable; and it was quiet, and Cousin Jim liked it. When later on electric lights replaced the gas, the room became more cheerful, and Cousin Jim enjoyed the adjustable standing lamp which enabled him to read while lying on the sofa.

George Richards Minot was born in this house at 188 Marlborough Street, Boston, on December 2, 1885. He was a delicate child, who caught every one of the childhood diseases and was quite sick with each. His health was never good. Pains in his legs and stomach troubled him from time to time, so that he spent a good deal of his childhood in bed, although, so far as I know, no definite diagnosis of a chronic disease was ever made.

Just why he was confined to bed so much is hard to say, but it is not surprising that his father's anxiety made the boy all the more conscious of any physical symptoms that he might have had. George's mother would not have insisted on so much rest in bed if the decision had been left to her, but her husband had been one of the pioneers in the new theories about the prevention and the early treatment of incipient pulmonary tuberculosis, and at the time of George's childhood he was a Visiting Physician to the Massachusetts General Hospital. Considering his knowledge, how could his wife express any doubts she might have about the management he prescribed? Since the doctor had seen a number of friends and relatives, as well as patients, die of tuberculosis, one must not blame him for taking extra care of his children, especially when his first-born was so tall and thin, like the typical candidate for the disease.

All matters of general health were important; chilling of the body was to be avoided at all costs. If it looked like rain, rubbers and raincoat were required, and if a boy wet his feet an immediate change of shoes and stockings was enforced.

Food was especially important in the Minot household; the boys must have the best of everything, prepared and served properly, and they *must* eat. "George, you must eat that — every bit of it!" How often did I hear this admonition!

This attention to food and to physical protection was destined to continue throughout George's life, but he led a fairly strenuous existence in spite of it. One can speculate that this early emphasis on food paved the way for George's great concern about the diet of his patients, and then about the relations between food and disease. But that is getting way ahead.

Influential in George's early life was his brother Henry's nurse, Mary McRae. She helped Mrs. Minot with all her children. She was a quiet, good-natured woman who had come from Prince Edward Island when she was barely out of her teens; she stayed with the Minots until she died in her eighties. She kept the house and she kept the boys — including me at times — in order.

My family lived in Milton all the year, and when I began to commute to school in Boston, Cousin Jim gave me a door key to 188, and I went in and out as I liked. When I was older, I kept my party clothes in a bureau drawer in the guest room, and Mary kept them clean and neat for me.

When George was sick, Mary was better than a nurse, for she understood the eccentricities of the whole family. She, too, did her bit in coaxing George to eat.

Most of the small boys in the Back Bay of Boston were sent to private schools, where the instruction and the environment were considered better than in the public schools. George was six years old when his mother first took him to Miss Fiske's School. Miss Fiske was an energetic, able woman of strong character, who each year introduced a new group of little boys and girls to the mysteries of the three R's. Her school was in a private house on Dartmouth Street, within easy walking distance of 188 Marlborough, and George went there for five years. Miss Fiske and her assistants gave him an excellent start so far as his education was concerned. Unfortunately, his poor health forced him to drop back a whole class.

In 1895, the Back Bay was still in the process of development. On Beacon and Marlborough Streets, and especially on Commonwealth Avenue nearby, new houses were building. The houses of that era were single dwellings, each for one family, tall and thin, four and often five stories high, built wall to wall with bay windows in front and back. There were only one or two apartment houses in the Back Bay then, and the very idea of a commercial enterprise like a shop in the neighborhood was frowned upon. The Vendome and the Victoria Hotels were the only exceptions in the area, and they came to be tolerated. The Somerset Hotel, beyond Massachusetts Avenue, was almost "out of town," and that was all right.

After school and on Saturdays, the boys played in one of the empty lots in the neighborhood, each lot being preëmpted by a special group. Each boy tended to play with his own friends, and the friends were not likely to mingle with outsiders. In this way, the children were somewhat like their parents, who, once established, developed a group of friends and then clung to it. The Back Bay was conservative, and its people all thought alike and had the same interests. The environment was secure; the world was pleasant, peaceful, and comfortable. The men were successful in their professions, but the women had little to do outside of their houses — or inside, for that matter, since young girls from Ireland or Nova Scotia made excellent servants and were glad to live and work in comfortable and secure homes even if the pay was small. The people of the Back Bay were inclined to spend their money cautiously: charities were not well organized and the needs of schools, colleges, and hospitals were not considered seriously. As for contributing money for research in science, engineering, or medicine, the possibilities were not even imagined at that time. Money could be spent, but there was no urge to give it away.

A few families had horses and carriages with coachmen, but when most people went out to dinner, or downtown to the theater, they hired a horse cab. Otherwise, people either walked or waited for the horsecar, which ran on Marlborough Street, back and forth from Massachusetts Avenue to Park Square.

The Back Bay was a dusty place. The streets were gravel, hard to keep in repair, and in dry weather every horse and team or carriage that went by raised dust. On windy days, great clouds of dust would rise spontaneously and come blowing down the street. Watering carts helped a little. Traffic was no problem, and small boys could cross the street without particular danger. In winter a good fall of snow was welcome, for the sleighing, especially on Commonwealth Avenue, was good, and on school-day afternoons we boys liked to jump on the back runner of the covered sleighs called "boobies." Ordinarily the coachman sitting up front on his open box could not see us crouching behind the body, but I remember the day when his long whiplash came around the side of the boobie and caught me across the face. After that our enthusiasm for punging waned a little.

When Miss Fiske's boys graduated, at about the age of twelve, they separated into two principal groups, one entering the Noble and Greenough School at 100 Beacon Street, the other going to the Volkmann School on Trinity Place, both in the Back Bay. These also were private schools. George entered the Volkmann School in 1896. In 1901, Mr. Volkmann built a new building for his school at 415 Newbury Street and I joined the school at that time, entering George's class.

At the Volkmann School, George was good in his studies and was promoted every year, but he was far from brilliant. His conduct was good; he did not have to stay after school either to make up deficiencies in his lessons or to multiply enormous numbers as a punishment.

Since Mr. Volkmann himself taught German, and since George was George, it is surprising that the boy had great difficulty with languages. Latin was hard for him. The puzzles of finding subject, object, and verb seemed complicated, and consequently French and German were difficult, too. The fact is that he entered college with a condition in German.

He was shy in school; he did not make friends quickly, but those he did make, stuck. He was still "delicate" — tall and much too skinny. His elders probably thought of him as a rather ungainly youth. At that age, it was physical and not intellectual prowess that counted. Although George had energy and a wiry endurance, he did not have the kind of strength and agility or the love of physical competition that appealed to our more athletic and aggressive classmates. Cousin Jim would not let him play football and did not want him to run on the track team. George did play a little baseball, however, and in his last year at Volkmann he played right field on the team and won his letter. He played hockey, too; we called it "shinny," and played it on week ends whenever there was ice on the ponds. No fancy equipment was necessary.

Every spring, most of the families in the Back Bay moved to the country. Many of them went to the North Shore, to places between Nahant and Gloucester where the southwest wind comes across the cold waters of Massachusetts Bay. Others, the Minots among them, went to the country to the southwest of Boston.

Cousin Bessie was the daughter of Mr. Henry Austin Whitney, a successful businessman, secretary of the Harvard Class of 1846, and — a fact that later pleased George — a trustee of the Massachusetts General Hospital. When Cousin Bessie married Cousin Jim in 1884, Mr. Whitney built for her the house at 188 Marlborough Street, and later she inherited a generous piece of the land that he had bought on the southern slope of Brush Hill in Milton, from which one had a good view of the Blue Hills, and on which she and Cousin Jim built a house. The house was bright and airy, with plenty of space around it. The gardens and stable were behind, near the road, and in front the land sloped gently down among big hardwood trees to a small pond made by a dam across the Mother Brook. George's maritime experiences began in this pond.

He and his cousin, Harry Whitney, who lived nearby, had built the *Puddle Duck*. She was only five feet long, but she could hold two boys and she didn't leak much. When she capsized one day, and George came home dripping, Cousin Jim was alarmed, but Cousin Bessie was amused, although she tried not to show it.

The group of children George played with in Milton was even more of a "closed corporation" than the Boston group, since they were all cousins. Besides Harry Whitney and me, there was Constance Zerrahn, whose mother was Cousin Bessie's sister. The Zerrahns also owned a house on the Whitney property.

In midsummer, the Minot family visited in Bar Harbor, Maine, with Cousin Jim's five sisters, "The Aunts." Their father, George Richards Minot (1813–1883), and his intimate friend and distant relative, Francis Minot Weld, had built in 1870 two houses just alike in "The Field" at Bar Harbor. The twin houses were simple frame cottages with wide verandas and a row of bedrooms upstairs. They contained none of the luxuries found in the lavish mansions built in

Bar Harbor later. The houses were placed on the waterfront, on a site from which one had magnificent views, of Frenchman's Bay and its rockbound islands in front, and of the mountains behind.

The new generation loved Bar Harbor as much as its elders had, and again the Minots played with the Welds. At the time of the Spanish-American War the children had an "army," of which George Minot, then thirteen, was general. The little Welds and Minots were one day lying face down in very prickly grass, pretending to be on a scouting party, when Marian Weld, aged eight, complained that they had been scouting long enough. "General Minot" said in a scathing tone: "You are very unpatriotic. Just think how our soldiers are suffering in Cuba." Marian relapsed into a mortified silence; George was a leader from the beginning.

When the children grew older, they played tennis on the court in front of the house, or went for walks in the deep woods or up the mountains, or sailed on the bay. Often they took long drives in a buckboard with a pair of horses, stopping in some lovely spot for a picnic. The summers in Bar Harbor were very pleasant.

When George was in his late teens, his health improved greatly. He had had hay fever since he was about twelve, with sneezing, itching eyes, and runny nose, beginning each summer in the middle of August and lasting until the first frost — the ragweed season. As time passed, the hay fever became worse. There was no good treatment in those days, but at Bar Harbor the symptoms were bearable, and on the water they were hardly noticeable. George's friend Bob Amory, whose father was also a doctor and a friend of Cousin Jim's, had a small Friendship sloop, the *Margery,* and George went cruising with him during several summers. George benefited enormously by the experience.

He and Bob learned much about charts, compasses, and buoys, about finding their way among the islands and in and out of harbors and coves. During one summer, they spent a total of thirty-five nights on the boat. It was good to be free from hay fever, but it was even better to escape from the family, from the petty anxieties about clothing and food. Bob Amory's simple, carefree, but effective management made a new way of life that was free and easy and pleasant, and gave George a self-confidence he needed badly.

George's illnesses had taught him to entertain himself. They had given him time to read and time to collect things. Postage stamps were an early interest, and the importance of little details of design, like the triangles in the corners of some American issues, taught him to observe and whetted his curiosity. His real interest, however, was in butterflies.

It is not clear how this interest began, but Cousin Jim approved of hunting and catching butterflies as a healthy exercise. He gave George books about butterflies and helped him to study them. He also gave him a cabinet in which to arrange and display his collection. I can remember looking over George's shoulder at the cabinet with a mixture of awe and curiosity. After a few years, each drawer held at least fifty specimens, each with its wings well spread and its body impaled on a pin. Even I could see that the specimens in each drawer were related one to the other. I believe that it was a fairly complete assembly of the common butterflies of New England. I know that George was quite proud of it; he would show the drawers to Harry Whitney and me — but he would warn us to be careful and not to touch them.

One of his best advisers about butterflies was our Cousin Charles Sedgwick Minot, who was the Professor of Histology and Human Embryology at Harvard Medical School. He was recognized all over the world as the authority in his field. When he came to call at Cousin Jim's house, George was glad, for it was easy to invite Cousin Charles to come up to his room and help him to classify some of the new specimens. The Professor liked to teach, and George was an excellent pupil, obviously keenly interested in his work. Cousin Charles also provided George with books about butterflies, and some years later he gave him the three handsome volumes of *Butterflies of North America,* by William H. Edwards.

George's knowledge of butterflies was very real, and the ease with which he could pick up and remember their tongue-twisting names was impressive to Harry Whitney and me. If we had only known then what we know now, Harry and I would have been wise to show a more critical interest, so that we in turn could have learned.

Partly on account of George's delicate health, Cousin Jim took him South for a week or two for several winters. In 1898 father and son went to Palm Beach, Florida, where the mother joined them later. There is an interesting letter from George to "The Aunts," describing the thrill of seeing ships of the United States Navy steaming southward not far off the shore, on their way to the Spanish War. On that trip, and on others to Kittrell, North Carolina, with Cousin Jim and a doctor friend, George brought back excellent specimens of butterflies, some quite different from those seen in Milton or Bar Harbor.

In the late autumn of 1900, when George was not quite fifteen, all the Minots went out to Santa Barbara, California, for the winter. The expedition was arranged chiefly for George. It seemed likely that if the boy could escape the New England winter and lead a healthy life out of doors in a warm, even climate for several months, his general condition would improve. Out in Santa Barbara he learned to ride a horse. In the spring of 1901 he was riding one day with his mother and father over the hills when he saw something that interested him so much that he wrote his first scientific paper about it. It was published in *Entomological News* for May 1902, under the title, "The Chrysalis of Melitaea Gabbi." [1] It reads in part:

> On April 5, 1901, I found a chrysalis of *Melitaea gabbi* hung to a cover of a paste board box, which was lying beside the road . . . [The place was] 1200 feet above sea level and . . . about eighteen miles from Santa Barbara, California.
>
> On April 9, 1901, at Monteceto, Santa Barbara . . . I watched a *Euchlae sara* variety *Reakirti* deposit an egg. It was about ten in the morning when I noticed this butterfly hovering round some of the common mustard; suddenly it alighted on a leaf and curving its abdomen round the leaf deposited an egg on the under side . . . On looking at it on April 10th [it was still there] . . . on . . . April 11th at nine o'clock . . . it was the same as before, but when I went back to look for it at half past eleven to take it into the house, I found the whole field of grain had been cut and the mustard plant, too, much to my sorrow.

Early in 1903, George published his second paper, this time a letter to the editor of the *Boston Evening Transcript,* Boston's best newspaper, which often contained items of scholarly interest. George was concerned about the damage caterpillars were doing to the trees of Boston; his letter was headed "The Tussock Moth Peril." [2] Here are two paragraphs:

It seems a pity that the City of Boston does not look after its shade trees better. Last spring the city had a few men go round with ladders and cutters and do some slow work in cutting off the egg clusters of the tussock moth (Orgyia Leucostigma). But the work amounted to nothing as there are as many eggs on the trees in most places this winter as last . . . When the men went round last spring, many worked diligently but as many more worked like snails and were very careless in their work. They would at times cut off twice as much of a branch as necessary and regardless of the tree would cut off branch and all in order to get a small egg cluster off . . .

It seems a shame all [the egg clusters] cannot be cleared away . . . If they are not . . . destroyed . . . the caterpillars will hatch and eat greedily the new leaves . . . After the caterpillar has grown to its full size, it spins a cocoon of dirty white color; it passes about fifteen days in the cocoon stage. Then the moth hatches and mates, the female laying her eggs upon the cocoon from which she hatched and covering them with a gummy substance. One female will lay a hundred eggs and more, sometimes less. The females are wingless and live only long enough to lay eggs, then die. The male has wings but has not the necessary organs with which to feed and lives like the female but a few days. After the moth hatches in June and has laid eggs, the caterpillars from these eggs hatch in a few days and feed till full grown, when they spin their cocoon and in a few days hatch into moths and this brood of moths lay the eggs which pass the winter in the egg stage and hatch in the spring. If these winter eggs are destroyed and a band of dendroline or the like be put around the tree trunk, so that no wandering caterpillar can get up to become a moth and lay eggs, the tree is safe from harm. The city apparently has given no thought to the consideration that they may get up the trunk.

This letter was written when George was only seventeen. It was based on his own reading and observation; he had not yet had any formal course in biology.

Even when he was grown up, George was always on the lookout for butterflies. Without warning he would rush off into the underbrush with his hat in hand, ready to capture an important specimen. In our school days, a favorite pastime in the spring was collecting moths at night. On our bicycles we would ride to the brightest street lamps on Blue Hill Avenue or Brush Hill Road in Milton. George would watch the moths and other insects for a while, and then he would make a sweep with his long-handled butterfly net and scoop in the one he wanted. I held the cyanide jar, which always seemed to me a mysterious and dangerous piece of equipment, and George would ease the moth into the lethal chamber. On warm evenings in May and June, when the frogs were croaking and the hylas were humming, these expeditions were very pleasant. If we wanted to sit on the stone wall and smoke a cigarette, there was no one to say us nay.

Lest the reader get the impression that young George was a sort of precocious genius, interested only in nature in general and in butterflies in particular, let me confess that he and Harry Whitney and I stole signs. We were an independent lot, and it was repugnant to us to read "No Trespassing," or better, "Trespassing or Fishing on this Property will be Prosecuted to the Full Extent of the Law." The town of Milton had a police force, with officers who patrolled at night on foot. In our Brush Hill section, the unhappy patrolman was supposed to cover an area about two miles long and about a mile wide. Officer Fallon in his Stanley Steamer, which was capable of real bursts of speed, was a much later development. Just why our officer was not provided with a bicycle I do not know, but one can see that it was not difficult for George and Harry and me to know where the cop was and when it was safe to remove the signs that were so offensive to us, and then to store them under the Whitneys' house. Dangerous work like this was exciting, and it was very enjoyable.

In February 1903, when George was seventeen, a dreadful calamity struck the Minot family. Cousin Bessie caught a bad cold and developed pneumonia. Young Doctor Edwin A. Locke, who had worked under Cousin Jim at the Boston Consumptives' Hospital, came to stay with the patient, and other doctors were called in. The best nurses were obtained, too, but in spite of everything that anyone could think of to do for her, the beloved lady died. Poor Cousin Jim was overcome by the tragedy; he had depended on his wife for encouragement in his work as well as for the management of his children and his home, and now she was gone. He never recovered from the blow of losing her, and for the rest of his life he wore black clothes and black ties. If before this he had been quiet and shy, without much sense of humor, he was really subdued afterwards. His five sisters did what they could to help him, but his loneliness was acute.

IN THE BEGINNING

He was a busy doctor of fifty, left in the prime of his life with three very active boys — George, seventeen, Jimmy, eleven, and Henry, seven — and alone responsible for their care and management. He was not strong physically, he was tired most of the time, and he had outside responsibilities in his hospital connections. Who was to play with his boys, to show them the love and affection that they needed? He did not know how to play. He wanted peace and quiet in the house; noise disturbed him. Although he was glad to help George with his stamps and butterflies, he was not sympathetic with games played on the floor with the rugs and the furniture pushed out of place. After Cousin Bessie died, there was not much laughter or fun in the house at 188 Marlborough Street. The Aunts came over frequently, but they were prim and proper maiden ladies older than their brother, too old for frolics.

On Sundays, the father and sons would go to the Aunts' for dinner or supper. The atmosphere in the big house at 245 Marlborough Street was pleasant enough, but it could not be called exciting. The boys must be dressed up, and usually on the way over Cousin Jim would warn them: "You will please behave yourselves; do you understand?"

To spend week ends in the country was more enjoyable, and beginning with our last years in school, George came often to stay at my father's house in Milton. He and I liked to go on long hikes through the Blue Hills Reservation. If we took our lunch with us, the day was even more pleasant, for then there was no hurry and we were independent and free. In the spring and fall we played golf, and at one time George was champion of the Hoosic Whisick Club. His score of 37 for the nine holes was a record. In school days, it was possible to catch the 2:15 train from the Back Bay Station and ride to Green Lodge, a whistle stop where the station at Route 128 is today. It was only a mile walk to the club and we had time for nine and sometimes eighteen holes of golf. After the game, my mother would send the carriage for us and we would spend the night in Milton.

In summer, my family went to Chappaquiddick, a good-sized island that lies opposite a curve in the shoreline of Martha's Vineyard to make the harbor of Edgartown, Massachusetts. Captain

Sandsbury made "Chappy" a wonderful place. My father had bought the house from him and then had arranged for the Captain to take care of it and of the Rackemann family.

Captain Sandsbury was a thickset little man, not over five feet four inches tall, quick of eye and hand. He had the shoulders of a stevedore and the forearms of a blacksmith. He had been around the Horn in a full-rigged ship. Primarily he was a sailor, but he was also a carpenter, painter, plumber, and gardener. His stubby pipe was a part of his costume. If we caught him without it and offered him a cigarette, he'd say, "No, thanks — got my pipe in my pocket."

He was friend and companion as well as keeper and guardian to my family for twenty-five years. When we boys came down in off-season, he was delighted. The first of these trips was in the Easter vacation of 1904, when George was eighteen and I was not quite seventeen; it was the first time we had been allowed to go off, free and independent, by ourselves. My account of the trip, which I kept in a special notebook, begins as follows:

April 1st, 1904. At about ten minutes before six a.m. I crawled out of bed at 188 Marlborough St. . . . and reached for the string leading down into George's room and pulled it. [The string went from my window down to George's window and was attached to several tin cans in his room.] . . . Cousin Jim had breakfast with us and helped us get under way. He made George take an umbrella . . . We left the house at 6:50 with our dress-suit cases and felt mighty comfortable. We took a car to Boylston Street and from there walked to the south terminal . . . The train started on time at 7:38 . . . I forgot to say that George left his umbrella at the newsstand, and so that did not bother us any more . . . At 8:00 just before we reached Brockton, my alarm clock, which I had put into my bag, went off and caused considerable excitement . . . When we got to Woods Hole it was raining hard — I supposed on account of that blessed umbrella.

At Woods Hole the rain turned out to be a real "northeaster."

After the roughest crossing I have ever experienced, we reached Cottage City [now called Oak Bluffs] . . . We Got our trunks there all right, they having been sent down . . . the day before.

Imagine taking enough clothes, boots, and coats to need a trunk for a ten-day trip!

Here is a sample of our daily activities:

"April 8, 1904. This morning the Captain came as usual at 7:45 and brought mail and paper. We had the alarm clock set for 8:00

and it managed to disturb me enough for me to get up at 8:15 and light the fire . . ."

My father had added a new kitchen to the house. It had windows on three sides, and was plenty big enough for two beds as well as the table, the stove, and the sink. The Glenwood range burned coal, and although it was temperamental at times, we learned to regulate the drafts and make it go. On that first trip, George and I slept in the kitchen, where it was warm and dry, but in later years, when we were joined by other boys, we found out that the regular beds upstairs were comfortable, even if in the first few minutes they felt a trifle chilly. The journal continues:

Pulling off George's blankets, I gave him a slap which roused him thoroughly . . . We had breakfast . . . and left the house at 9:05, having put some dry shoes and stockings, some chocolate, and George's camera into a bag . . . The wind was S × E and so we had to beat in the sailboat all the way to the South Beach . . . We struck a place where the clams were quite thick. Captain dug 3 pails to our one . . . We got 30 odd little necks . . . Back at home the Captain suggested that we try some clams done in another way — fried — so I helped Captain cook the clams while George wrote letters . . . The clams were a success, I having three helpings of them . . .

April 10, 1904. According to our agreement of the night before, we set the alarm clock for 6: a.m. As I had put several tin pans under it, it made more effect on us and we got up soon after. We had breakfast and were under way [walking] by 8:20 after taking our lunch with us . . . We arrived [at the Cape Poge Lighthouse] at 10:59 . . . The keeper — Mr. Eldridge — was very nice and asked us to come in and get warm. They were evidently glad to see human faces: gave us letters to mail for them . . . [On the way back] we sat down to lunch . . . under a very old and knotty cedar and ate it . . . George in opening the water bottle burst the cork, and as he had to push it in, he thought that he had dirtied the water and so refused to drink any . . . We reached home about 3:00 p.m. . . . Vegetable soup, beefsteak, guava jelly, corn, potatoes, pickles, triscuit, apple-pie and doughnuts, coffee a la demi-tasse for dinner.

Since our first trip to Chappy was so successful, we went there for every Easter vacation through college and medical school, taking friends along, six or eight of us at a time. We called ourselves the "Edgartown High School."

Staple food like canned goods, sugar, and tea was sent down ahead of time from S. S. Pierce's store — the standard source of good food in Boston — and when one time we asked the Captain, "Did you get any express packages for us?" he replied, "Yes, by gorry, there was a barrel and a box and another box and a leetle box." How George Minot loved to repeat that line! If the Captain recognized a case of beer waiting for us before those later vacations, he never "let on" to the folks at home.

George Minot loved his food, but he did not know much about cooking it. When my mother told me about the soup kettle — how the bones of steak, the carcasses of chicken, and meat remnants of almost any kind should be put in a pot with a few onions and carrots and some salt and pepper and should be allowed to simmer on the back of the stove almost indefinitely — the expression "Save it for soup" became a watchword. (Incidentally, there are some advantages in having a coal stove!) On the next day the contents of the kettle would be passed through a clean dishcloth, and the liquid set outside to cool. When the crust of fat was lifted off and the thick, usually jellied, liquid was reheated, it was good soup — to my taste, it was wonderful soup. George, however, was not so sure; he had seen the preparations and was skeptical about using the remnants, which he would have thrown in the garbage can. Later he agreed that the soup was wholesome after all and that it tasted all right.

During the summer after we had graduated from the Volkmann School, George came to visit me at Chappy. We hit upon the idea of walking to Gay Head, a distance of at least twenty-five miles across Martha's Vineyard. The plan was to camp for the night in West Tisbury, about ten miles away, and then on the next day to leave our equipment, walk the fifteen miles to Gay Head, turn around, and come back to the same camp.

We collected a tent, blankets, rubber sheets, a lantern, a pail, extra sweaters and shoes, a saucepan, and enough food for three days, and rowed across the harbor to Ed Smith's landing. The bulky items were tied to a long pole carried between us. On the way across the "Martha's Vineyard Desert" to West Tisbury, the pole became heavier and heavier, the blankets in rolls across our shoulders hotter and hotter.

In midafternoon, the sight of a house was wonderful, and when the old man there saw that we were not entirely crazy, he laughed with us. When he said that we could set up our tent in his pine grove and draw water from his well, what a relief that was! A friend in need is a friend indeed, and he was it.

On the next day, our hike to Gay Head, with our baggage left behind us, was easy enough. At Menemsha Bight, a fisherman was suspicious at first, but he set us across the creek. On the beach below the colored cliffs of Gay Head we swam and ate our sandwiches. The walk back was easy, too, and we reached camp when the sun was still high. Then a remarkable thing happened. In spite of all that walking, it was George who said, "Why not go home right now?"

We gave all the food to our new friend, so that the pole was not quite so heavy and the blanket rolls did not feel quite so hot. We did the ten miles in less than three hours. I was never so tired in my life, but how George survived the day, walking a total of roughly forty miles, is hard to explain. He wrote me later, "We really had a bully time and good experience going to Gay Head: wish we could do it again." Even in retrospect, it was a successful venture.

The fact is that we did do it again, and in the very next summer, when Tommy Clark, our classmate, went with us. He remembers the expedition to this day, and his memory is a pleasant one, free of any resentment for the physical fatigue that he endured.

From this, it is quite evident that at nineteen George Minot had improved in health tremendously. Besides energy, we both had something our friends did not have: we had the ability to enjoy the scenery, whether in town or country, and to observe interesting things as we went by.

When that summer was over, George and I planned to enter Harvard College. Of course! Our relatives and friends had gone there; it was the logical and natural thing to do after graduation from school. No alternative was suggested or considered. The only problem had concerned the examinations for admission and whether we could pass them. The examinations were divided into two parts: Preliminaries at the end of the Second Class (junior year) and Finals when we graduated in the First Class. What a grueling period the examinations were! Preliminaries consisted of seven examinations taken during three days, and we crammed hard both before and during that dreadful experience. Finals were harder, with the same subjects in advanced, instead of elementary, status. The list included advanced Latin, French, and German — two hours of each — solid geometry, physics, and finally, logarithms and trigonometry. I saw the questions again the other day and could not answer them. However, since, except for George's German, we passed everything, Mr. Volkmann and his men must have taught us well.

2

Harvard College

In September 1904, George, almost nineteen, became a freshman at Harvard College, where he lived in a single room in Apley Court. The dormitories on or near Mount Auburn Street in Cambridge — Apley, Dunster, Claverly, Russell, Westmorely, and the new Ridgely — were large buildings built for this purpose and owned by private interests quite separate from Harvard College. The area was referred to sometimes as the "Gold Coast" because the rooms and suites were more luxurious and expensive than the rooms in the College Yard. Most of George's school friends lived in the area. When Mr. A. Lawrence Lowell became President of Harvard in 1912, he interested Mr. Edward Harkness in helping him to organize the new Houses along the Charles River, and the student body became more diversified. Most of the former Gold Coast became Adams House.

In 1904, I was considered too young for college life, so I stayed on at the Volkmann School, anticipating several courses that gave me advanced credit. I went out to Cambridge a number of times, but as a schoolboy I felt very much out of place. George was busy and appeared to be enjoying himself with friends; most of them were schoolmates from Boston, but new friends gradually increased in number. He ate most of his meals at a table in a boarding house with a dozen or so classmates. The group was organized to provide a place to eat in company that was friendly and reasonably satisfactory. There were many of these "tables" in Cambridge; they were all temporary, without the formal aspects of a club. The food was fair, but for George it was never good enough. It did not take more than a friend's suggestion to make him decide to dine at the Harvard Union, where the food was better, even if a little more expensive, or, better still, to go in town for a real dinner at home or in a restaurant.

George was slow to make new friends. This was partly because of his health and physique, for at that age athletic ability was important. He was too thin, and he thought of himself as far from rugged, although he looked well and obviously had a wiry endurance. There were times when he felt inferior and insecure. He was skeptical about new people, wondering subconsciously what they might do to him. He would ask one of his Boston cronies: "Who is this man? Did you ever see him before? Where does he come from? What do you know about him?" Some sort of label had to be attached before George would accept the new man. It was hard for him to size up a new acquaintance in a short time; he hesitated to take the man at his face value, especially since he was the same age as George. Later, when his friends seemed to like the newcomer, George was ready to "play ball" with him. In his freshman year, George was not what one might call a good mixer. It was not until he joined his "final" club in sophomore year that he established any new and lasting friendships with his classmates.

George went to the theater frequently, often bringing a friend or two to dine with his father at "188" before the play. There were no movies in 1905. Travel from Cambridge to Boston was by street car over Massachusetts Avenue. On real occasions, when they stayed in town for oysters and beer after the show, he and his friends would ride back to Cambridge in Tom Kelly's hack, with the old nag trotting as fast as his tired legs would allow.

Week ends were spent in the country, often at my father's house in Milton, and that meant golf or another hike in the Blue Hills, depending on the time of year. When the sleighing was good, it was fun to take the big double-runner — it would be called a bobsled today — and go coasting on the roads on those beautiful moonlight nights when the air was clear and cold and still. It was not often that we had to wait for a horse and sleigh to get out of the way.

Under the elective system, the choice of courses required careful thought. With his father a doctor, his Cousin Charles Minot a professor in the Medical School, and other relatives on both sides interested in medicine, George knew that his blood had a medical tinge to it. He talked often about becoming a doctor, but it was a nebulous goal, never clearly defined. He liked all the biological sciences, anyway, and since further knowledge of them might help as a preparation for medicine, he included some in his schedule, especially in the later college years.

In freshman year, he took five courses. Almost everybody took Government 1 and listened to Mr. A. Lawrence Lowell, a delightful gentleman and obviously a distinguished person who was later to be President of Harvard. George took History 1A and English A ("Prescribed English"). In the first half year, he took Zoology 1 under Professor George H. Parker, with his little brown goatee and his interesting lectures; and then Botany 1 under Professor George Lincoln Goodale for the second half year. It is not surprising that George got a B in zoology. In botany he got only a C, but the course dealt more with the classification of plants than with their structure and functions. Since he had entered college with the condition in German, he was required to take the elementary course to work it off. He did not like German and he did not like the course. The fact is that he didn't like languages.

In sophomore year, life was much easier. George came back to college with many friends, and the difficulties of meeting new men were distinctly fewer. College was not so new; the way around was familiar; he felt much more at home. In his sophomore year he roomed in Claverly Hall, another building on the Gold Coast, with Tommy Clark, an old friend from the Volkmann School. This was a year of social activity in college, and studies were of only secondary concern, except that one had to pass the latter in order to enjoy the former. It was the year of election to clubs.

In those days, there were six clubs at Harvard that were "final," in the sense that no man who belonged to one club could belong to any of the others. George's and my final club was the Owl Club, which became almost our second home. We ate most of our meals there, and came to know intimately a group of men who became our close friends for all time. The group had similar backgrounds, habits, interests, and ideals, and George felt particularly secure on this common ground. His part, however, was not prominent; he never held an official position in any college club.

There were other clubs that were not final. In sophomore year election and initiation to the "Dickey" (D.K.E.) was an important goal. The Dickey was a unique organization. It was a horizontal selection of men from all the final clubs, with a few from outside any club. Most of George's friends were elected sooner or later. The initiation was strenuous, for from one Thursday night to the next the week was a dreadful experience. The neophyte was tormented in every way. He was obliged to learn lines of poetry, the lists of the Presidents of the United States and the Presidents of Harvard College, and he must be able to recite these at any hour of the day or night. He must wear his coat inside out, have only sneakers on his feet, leave off his hat and overcoat, regardless of the weather, and run everywhere and never walk. In the evening the rituals were severe. Each morning the poor fellow must be up at six to deliver newspapers to his list of "wake-ups," and he must be ready to close the window, run errands, or even sing a song.

This initiation has been abandoned now, but in some ways it was not such a bad experience, for it taught every man to know his own strength, to find out that he could get by without much sleep, that he could learn things quickly if it was really necessary, and that he could adapt himself both physically and mentally if he had to. George Minot stood up well under this grueling — much better than he had expected. Having survived, he felt more secure than before. He had taken a severe test and had passed it, and in so doing he had been forced into contact with men in other classes, with men who lived in other dormitories, and with men who came from many different places. He found that he could meet them more easily than he had expected and that they were not so bad after all. He had proved to himself that he "belonged."

In sophomore year, George's social life expanded toward Boston. A series of "coming out" balls, each given by a generous lady of society to introduce her daughter, was held in the Louis XIV Ballroom in the Hotel Somerset. On almost every Friday night, George and I and most of our friends were invited to one of these balls, and quite often we went. The Big Ballroom was a handsome place, and the lovely ladies, with their dresses of satin and lace, were matched by the gentlemen in white ties and tails, always with white kid gloves, and usually with flowers in their buttonholes. When Mr. Gott, the bandmaster, had imbibed just the right amount of champagne, his playing of the Strauss waltzes set us all in motion. Dancing became irresistible. About midnight, supper was served at the tables in the Somerset dining room. There was clear soup, scrambled eggs or perhaps creamed chicken or lobster, and then fancy ice cream with spun sugar around it. The champagne was wonderful, and the food and drink made us ready to dance again. After supper there was often a cotillion, with favors varying from cardcases to necklaces, from horse whips to tinsel wands. As we started home, usually long after three o'clock in the morning, the cup of hot beef broth that was handed to us at the door went to the right spot.

George enjoyed these parties. He liked to dance even if he didn't dance easily. He knew one or two girls well, but his approach and his manner were distinctly formal. At that age, there was little contact with girls except in the Somerset Ballroom and at one or two smaller dances given in private homes. Dinner parties before the balls were helpful and resulted in more security for both the boys and the girls later in the evening.

One day in the spring, when the ball was even better than usual, George and I stayed until dawn. The sun was coming up as we walked down Marlborough Street. A milkman was making his rounds, but he stopped his horse to sell us two quarts of milk. To think of George Richards Minot, inquisitive physician, sitting on the curbstone on Marlborough Street in his dress suit and patent-leather shoes, silk hat on the back of his head and his collar and shirt all caved in, drinking a whole quart of milk on the spot, is almost impossible — but I was there!

Sophomore year did have its serious side. The courses George took included Economics 1, which was not very appealing, since commerce, exchange, and currency were not in his line. Chemistry 1, given by Professor Charles L. Jackson, was more interesting, although at that time the relation of chemistry to biology was not appreciated. George was not good in the laboratory; he was clumsy with his hands. If the directions said to add a few drops, George was apt to dump in a quantity and so carry the reaction too far and spoil its clear-cut result.

History 27 was one of George's strong subjects, for through it he met Mr. Roger B. Merriman, who seemed to return a little of George's admiration. "Frisky" Merriman had been seen in the

Somerset Ballroom, and to George that was greatly in his favor, like a good label on a bottle of wine. Mr. Merriman's teaching made George interested in European history; I know because George used to tell me about it.

Everyone had to have one or two "snap courses" to smooth out the general average. George selected landscape architecture and anthropology, and did well in both; in fact, he was pleased to find that the study of man's early beginnings and the history of his intellectual and physical development were much more interesting than he had anticipated.

In Junior year he lived in Russell Hall with Tommy Clark and A. William Reggio, another old friend from the Volkmann School. Reggio was destined to go to medical school with us, and his tastes for the biological sciences were somewhat similar to George's. Both Clark and Reggio had walked with us on day trips through the Blue Hills. Clark was a small man, but bright, active, and strong; Reggio was bigger. Both were good company.

When George studied anthropology again, it was because he liked it, and he received honors in the one and one-half courses that he took under Dr. William C. Farabee and Dr. Roland B. Dixon. Besides another history course and another economics course on transportation, he elected Chemistry 3 and Social Ethics 1.

Chemistry 3 consisted chiefly of laboratory work. The student was given a sample of queer-looking material, usually in powder form, and was asked to find out what was in it. If we followed the system of qualitative analysis, the technique was not difficult, and the course was pleasant — chiefly, I suppose, because it was so "practical."

Social Ethics 1 was reputed to be a "snap course," but again it held more interest than George expected. Furthermore, it was given by the Reverend Francis Greenwood Peabody, a friend of George's father. Mr. Peabody himself was the father of Dr. Francis W. Peabody, who was to become important in George's medical career. George enjoyed the course. The story of how people lived and how they behaved toward one another, the composition and the workings of society, fitted well with his studies in anthropology, and the science of the subject appealed to and enhanced his sympathetic feelings for his fellow men. The thesis George wrote was entitled "The

New Social Work at the Massachusetts General Hospital," and in it he described the new Department of Social Service, founded there by Dr. Richard C. Cabot in November 1905, with the help of Miss Ida B. Cannon.

As a senior, George was still more secure. He lived in Randolph Hall with Edward Wigglesworth; Clark and Reggio had moved. The Owl Club provided a good base, and his friendships there developed rapidly and soundly. He had also made many friends outside the club, so that his life was richer. In this year, his courses were selected with much greater care, and, except for a course in history, they were all in science.

Botany 2, a half course under Professor Roland Thaxter, dealt with fungi, beginning with the ferns and mosses and going down the scale of complexity to that enormous group of unicellular organisms, the molds, which make beer and wine ferment, which produce the green color in Roquefort cheese, and which mildew the sails on boats. At that time, Professor Thaxter, working in his dingy, moldy laboratory, seemed to be struggling with useless knowledge, but today we have penicillin and other mold-produced antibacterial substances, and we learn that molds alone can cause a number of human diseases, so that, as President Lowell was wont to predict, the "useless knowledge" has suddenly become of the greatest practical importance.

Chemistry 2 was a series of lectures by Professor Henry A. Torrey on organic chemistry. I took it with George. We enjoyed the formulae, but now in retrospect it seems a shame that there was no laboratory work to demonstrate the basis for the symbols that Professor Torrey used. George helped Bill Reggio and me to understand why it is that alcohol really is ethyl hydroxide with the formula C_2H_5OH.

Chemistry 15, a half course given by Professor Lawrence J. Henderson, concerned the chemistry of the animal body and was "pretty deep stuff," as the undergraduates called it. Dr. Henderson was a stoutish man with sparse red hair and a reddish beard. He talked in a high squeaky voice, which amused us at first. He was destined to be important later on to both George and me. In Chemistry 15 it was easy to see that Dr. Henderson had hold of a principle that was important for the preservation of normal chemical relations in the blood, and thus for the welfare of the whole body. George got an A in the course.

Zoology 2, under Dr. William E. Castle, dealt with the morphology of animals, and George absorbed it all. Likewise, the course in physiology given by Dr. Eugene A. Darling was almost old stuff, including the dead cats that were pulled out of the jar of alcohol formalin for us to examine. Mining 16, George's last science course, under Professor Edward D. Peters, was supposed to be, and was, a "snap course."

In his senior year George received a straight A in every one of his subjects, a remarkable performance, and that made his total record so good that "Cum Laude" was added to his degree of A.B. I did not know about these good marks until recently when, with a little difficulty, I obtained permission to look at the official record. Why did I not know before? Granted the lack of respect for scholarship at Harvard in that decade, I would still have been pleased to tell George if I had obtained all A's. His reticence was remarkable. In later years, George received many awards and prizes for his wonderful work. He did talk about his Nobel prize, for that had been announced in the daily papers, but there was hardly a word about the lesser prizes. George was modest about these things.

In his four years at Harvard College, George Minot's personality had developed enormously. He had caught on to the value of knowledge and the methods of obtaining it. He not only could absorb, but he could classify and digest the material that was presented; it meant something to him. Meantime, he had become less shy, much more approachable, and ready to meet people on a common ground. He learned to look at the good side of life instead of being skeptical about those appearances and impressions that were not immediately favorable.

He learned another thing, something that was not appreciated by most of the college students of his day until many years after their graduation: that universities are among the most important institutions in the world, and that the teachers in them are chosen in large part because they are scholars who have contributed to the knowledge of their subjects. These professors are distinguished men who are attracted to the university by the opportunity to learn still more. The material facilities appeal to them, but the hope of association with other scholars of their own character appeals still more. George Minot was not slow to realize that such men as Mr. Lowell, Dean Briggs, and Mr. Merriman were superior men, worthy of great respect, and therefore of close attention. For him it was a privilege to attend their lectures and to hear them discuss their subjects.

He appreciated the fact that Professor Charles L. Jackson had played a part in developing the periodic table of the chemical elements. He realized that Dr. Henderson was working on an important proposition — that the blood plays a major role in maintaining the balance between acids and bases, and that the transport of oxygen, on the one hand, and of carbon dioxide, on the other, is related to the changes in this balance. The recognition of scholars and the appreciation of the atmosphere which is the University are new ideas that take time for the young student to grasp. This atmosphere appealed to George at the beginning; he enjoyed it always. Harvard did much for him.

In the spring of 1906, in George's sophomore year, Cousin Jim bought the *Dorel,* a lovely gaff-rigged cutter with a single head sail. She was a beautifully designed and beautifully built little ship — thirty feet long at the water line and forty-five feet over-all. She drew seven feet of water and this, together with her generous beam, gave her excellent stability, so that she felt solid and substantial. She was in no sense a racing yacht, but she could sail well enough to make good time even when beating against the wind. Because she had no engine, plans for a cruise on the *Dorel* were bound to be interesting in their uncertainty.

Her main cabin had a bunk built under the deck on each side, and under each bunk there was a transom that pulled out to make two other bunks, almost as comfortable. Forward of a partition was the galley with a sink, an icebox, and a shipmate range burning coal briquettes. Forward of the mast and the end of the cabin house was the fo'castle, with two pipe berths and lockers underneath.

Cousin Jim was fortunate to obtain the services of Captain Alfred Pettee and of Al Farnum. Captain Pettee, a strong, well-built man in his late forties, came from Isle au Haut, Maine. He had lived on the coast of Maine all his life, and he knew the sea. Cousin Jim could trust him to take care of his boys; he knew that with the Captain to guide them and guard them they would be safe and they would learn a lot.

Al Farnum was the cook. He had learned his trade in the old coasting schooners that carried coal down East to Maine and brought lumber and granite back to New York and Boston. It was a luxury to have a professional cook on such a small boat, but George and his brothers were to be cruising during most of the summer, and Cousin Jim believed that good meals were worth having regardless of what they might cost.

For seven summers, the *Dorel* sailed up and down the coast from Marblehead to Bar Harbor, with occasional extra cruises west to the Harvard-Yale crew races in New London or east to Passamaquoddy Bay and New Brunswick.

To be invited to go cruising on the *Dorel* was a thrill; George's friends enjoyed it as much as did George himself. The coast of Maine is ideal for cruising. The mouths of many rivers and the great number and variety of islands encourage exploration of those little coves and harbors which the chart shows to have deep water and to be sheltered from the sea and wind. The quiet passages between islands make a pleasant contrast to the open bays.

It is fun to land at the town wharf in a new place, and to walk up the village street to find the post office and the general store at the crossroads. One learns about the price of butter and sugar, lemons, eggs, and fresh vegetables, if any, and especially of meat. Cruising teaches other things besides the handling of sails, the function of lighthouses and buoys, and the use of chart, compass, and parallel rulers.

George had friends in many ports, especially in North Haven and in Bar Harbor, and he could stay for a day or two or move on as the spirit moved him.

A number of incidents stand out, all recorded in the log book that George kept so carefully. I was on board once when we sailed all night from Marblehead to North Haven. My watch began shortly before sunrise — what an experience! I shall never forget it!

George liked New Brunswick, for not many people cruised so far to the eastward. He wanted to explore the shores of Passamaquoddy Bay. He was delighted to anchor one night inside the mouth of the Magaguadavic (pronounced "magadavey") River, where the fresh water made the barnacles drop off — or so the Captain said. And then there was the time when he and Orville Rogers, our classmate in medical school, and I got lost in the woods and had to walk back by the road to the cove where the boat lay — a distance of nine miles!

The *Dorel* put into Bar Harbor occasionally, and each time it did, there was a tremor of excitement in the Minot and Weld houses there. One can picture the Aunts standings on their piazza with field glasses, taking turns looking out to sea. When in the late afternoon the ship drifted in past the breakwater, the word would pass: "Here comes George!" Soon the boys would row ashore and come through the hole in the hedge, to be greeted with affection by the ladies and to enjoy a dinner that was a feast.

All during his senior year in college, George had been thinking and talking about medical school, but neither the thought nor the talk was very serious. I finished my college course at the same time as George, because I had been admitted to Harvard with extra credits. At the end of college in 1908, George and I were even in our years of academic standing.

Almost every time George and I came together, our talk included the question of medical school. We had both fulfilled the requirements for admission: we were about to receive our A.B. degrees and we had passed the required courses in chemistry. If we wanted to go to the Harvard Medical School, all we had to do was to walk in and register. That last, however, was such a vital step that it was hard to be sure that we wanted to take it. It is interesting that in our last year in Harvard College Cousin Charles Minot had hinted to our families that microscopes would make very acceptable graduation presents for us young "biologists," and he had said that he would be glad to select the proper instruments. When he advised this, he actually said nothing about medical school, but our families caught the idea. George and I were very pleased with our new toys.

In the spring of George's senior year, there was no hurry about coming to any decision. Nothing need be done about it then — or in the summer either, for that matter. The only deadline ahead was the day of actual registration. Another question was more important: would George Minot go to Europe in the summer with his classmates, Edward Wigglesworth, H. Webb Hyde, and Edward M. Stone? As the boys talked about it, the idea seemed better and better. George's father thought well of it, and that encouraged George. The trip was one more thing to think about, in addition to the final examinations and the plans concerned with graduation at Commencement on June 18, and so the thoughts and discussions about Europe postponed still longer the necessity for deciding about medicine. George would have made the itinerary, the tickets, and the hotel reservations into a series of complex problems if his three traveling companions had not made the details easy to execute.

In June, everything happened at once. Class Day, and the Spread at Beck Hall, offered a chance to return some of the hospitality of Boston Society, and the invitations had to be sent out. The Harvard-Yale baseball game attracted old graduates, and there were a luncheon and dinner at the Owl Club.

What George should take to Europe in the way of baggage and clothes was by no means a casual question. Should he include shirts of flannel as well as of cotton, and if so, how many? This problem required real discussion, and then in the middle of the preparations, George had a cold with bronchitis and trouble with his ear, which used up three valuable days. After Class Day and up to the time of sailing on June 30, George's life was hectic, to say the least.

On Saturday, June 27, when I was in Chappaquiddick for the summer, George wrote me an interesting letter:

> I have been talking over in the last few nights with Papa and others about what in Hell to do next winter, and especially the question of the M.D. school. I wish I knew. I may appear there yet if I get urged enough, yet I don't like the idea of being a freshman all over again and another four years of "exams." It remains to see what happens, and that's the worst part because it seems from what various people say that perhaps it is the place for me to go.

When we face a difficult decision, we like to have someone confirm our suppressed desires — to talk us into it — and so to share a little of the responsibility in case the choice turns out to be wrong. George, in particular, depended on the support and approval of others, and without it he was unhappy. He wrote me from the R.M.S. *Saxonia,* four days out to sea: "Well, maybe and maybe not I shall appear out to Longwood [the Harvard Medical School] in the autumn — Do write something about it — It is hard to think over such a plan with no one to constantly discuss the matter with me."

In Paris, the boys saw "everything." George's letters spoke of restaurants and top hats, the Louvre, and the prices of food and drink, and added that he was still worried about what to do in the fall. In Interlaken, he complained that the others were less energetic than he, and that he went out without them to see the sights. In Switzerland the party split up, Minot and Wigglesworth going to Venice and Milan, and Hyde and Stone going to Zermatt to climb the Matterhorn — and they did climb it! In Germany the four were reunited, and George wrote me about picture galleries and microscopes. In Berlin, the party split again, Hyde and Wigglesworth going off to London, and Minot and Stone exploring Copenhagen and Sweden before returning to meet the others back in Berlin. George wrote:

> You speak of your very healthy life and it makes me pretty envious . . . This traveling life is about as unhealthy as can be . . . I suppose I am just ruining my health with the continual pint [of wine] at supper and a few beers here and there . . . I hope to gain health in the U.S.A. I have indigestion at times . . . There is not a doubt if I was healthier now or even had been all my life, I would appear in Longwood in the autumn, but my nervous makeup plus never being very strong is a big hindrance & it is the one thing in the way to do for my life work what interests me . . . but it is hell to know how with my constitution I would get along. I think it over once a day & can't decide and who . . . will decide if I don't. When I get home and have decided to go, I will be told I am not strong enough and so I try not to think about it and then it won't be such a disappointment.

This letter shows what really was in George's heart. He did want to go to medical school — "to do for my life work what interests me" — and it was anxiety about his health that stood in the way of his final decision. The psychologist can explain how the "confession" was made in a moment of depression.

A month later, when he wrote to say that he was home, the same uncertainty was still troubling him: "I am up in the air in the worst way about the Medical School and the winter. It looks as if there would be a big lot of talking done in the next week."

Up to Saturday, September 26 — and that was only five days before the opening of medical school — neither George nor I had actually committed himself. That night I saw George for the first time since June. I dined at the Minots' Milton house and stayed late. To say that we had much to talk about is putting it mildly. On Sunday, George and I went to a tea at Cousin Charles Minot's house, and even then we were not definite in assuring our professor cousin that we would become members of his course the following week. That night, however, I telephoned to George, and I can still recall the conversation:

"I'll go if you'll go."

"All right, I'll go, too. You are sure that you will go?"

That settled it. On Monday there were chores and errands in town, with time enough to go out to Cambridge to watch football practice, and then on Tuesday morning George, Bill Reggio, and I went to Cambridge together, they to get their A.B. degrees, I to get my certificate saying that I could graduate next year with the Class of 1909. Although my diary does not say so, I presume that we had to secure the additional paper which would certify that our college courses had included the physics and chemistry the Harvard Medical School required. Armed with these credentials, we returned to the Medical School and signed on — "and That is That," as George remarked.

3

Harvard Medical School

The Harvard Medical School opened on Thursday, October 1, 1908, with a new incoming class of only sixty-five men — about one-half of the school's capacity of one hundred twenty-five. The reason for the small number was that in 1901 President Eliot had recommended to the Faculty of Medicine that all candidates for admission must have obtained the degree of Bachelor of Arts and also must show evidence of knowledge of physics and chemistry. The new standards became effective in 1905, and they discouraged many young men who had been led to believe that medicine was easy to learn and that its practice offered a pleasantly lucrative if not leisurely way of life. President Eliot's decree took away all thought of ease in the Medical School.

It is hard now to believe that in 1908 the Harvard Medical School was actively seeking prospective students. There was no need to screen the candidates to look for the best men. Every man who had a degree and a knowledge of chemistry was more than welcome. For our class sixty-five men were taken; the administration would have been glad to receive twice that number. Those who were unfit or poorly qualified would drop out as soon as dissection of the dead human body was started in the course in anatomy. That course was — it still is — an excellent and automatic eliminator of the unfit.

Today, forty years later, the limit of one hundred twenty-five men is still necessary, on account of laboratory space, and applications for these places pour in at the rate of over twelve hundred per year. Each candidate must imagine himself as standing in a line of ten men, and he must be so impressive in his personality and his aptitude, in his extracurricular achievements as well as in his college marks, that he will be the one in ten to be selected. No longer can the student hesitate or keep postponing his decision to enter the Medical School; he must make a formal application a year ahead of time. His credentials will be scrutinized with the greatest care, for to make the best doctor the best material is none too good.

In our day, the Harvard Medical School and the Johns Hopkins Medical School were considered to be the best in the country. This was not because the list of subjects taught was different from that in other schools; it was because in these two schools the professors were outstanding men who were trying hard to learn for themselves more about the fundamentals of medical science; they were seeking new knowledge, and as a result their attitudes were enthusiastic and their teaching was stimulating to all the young men who came under them. The reputations of Harvard and of Hopkins were beginning to develop, but not yet enough to draw many students from a distance. Most of the students in our class came from New England, although only a few came from Harvard College. The Medical School was still a local institution.

At 10 A.M. on Thursday, October 1, the sixty-five young men who had been admitted met together for the first time in Room 205 of the Administration Building, where Dr. Charles M. Green gave a lecture on manners. He reminded us that we had been "admitted to the company of educated men," as President Eliot had told us when he awarded our A.B. degrees, and we were supposed to act like men — like gentlemen, no less. Good manners, which mean courtesy and thought for others, were to be cultivated. Honesty and sincerity are implicit in the profession of medicine. We were to conduct ourselves with dignity. We could smoke in certain laboratories but never in lectures, and we must never smoke in a hospital. The nurses were students like ourselves; we were to have no contact with them except as it concerned the welfare of patients. Finally, our dress was important. At all times the doctor must be clean as to his person and his clothes. More than one has lost his patient because his hands and fingernails were dirty. Dr. Green did us a little good, probably, but we did not take all of his talk too seriously at that time.

In the first half of the first year the curriculum prescribed anatomy every morning and histology — our microscopes were appreciated — every afternoon. On our second day, Dr. Thomas Dwight, Parkman Professor of Anatomy, gave his first lecture in anatomy. He was an elderly gentleman, small in stature, with a rather large head and a full white beard that often almost, but not quite, touched the specimen he was demonstrating. His eyes were bright, his talk was cheerful, and he made a rather dry subject as interesting as possible. Each morning at nine he lectured and demonstrated for an hour.

Dr. Dwight was the direct successor to Dr. Oliver Wendell Holmes. During the years when Dr. Holmes had been giving the lectures in anatomy, Dr. Dwight had been giving a course of supplementary lectures in topographical anatomy. A year after Dr. Holmes resigned in 1882, Dr. Dwight was appointed to the Parkman Professorship. He had introduced the making and study of frozen sections of the human body. We young men did not know about this until later, but we could see quite easily that Dr. Dwight was an authority in his subject.

Dr. John Warren, son of Dr. J. Collins Warren and grandson of the Dr. John C. Warren who with Dr. James Jackson founded the Massachusetts General Hospital, was Assistant Professor of Anatomy. He gave the lectures on the anatomy of the nervous system. He was a great big man, at least six feet four inches tall, with a pince-nez eyeglass tethered by a long black ribbon. He was heavy in body and speech, devoid of humor, and he appeared to be pleased with his own recitation.

Dr. David Cheever was quite different. His talk was friendly and helpful. He "demonstrated" to us in small sections, and gave us short reviews on Saturday mornings. Each of us was given a box of bones to study as he read his anatomy books.

In the afternoons at two, Cousin Charles S. Minot, James Stillman Professor of Comparative Anatomy, aided by Dr. John Lewis Bremer, gave us lectures in histology and embryology. Cousin Charles talked well, and since most of the embryology that he taught us was based upon his own original observations, he made a complex subject interesting and understandable. His neckties amused us; they were of bright colors, red, green, blue, even pink and yellow, and always plain, and he tied them in a large knot. He was delighted when later on we showed him a list of his ties and the times when he wore them. It was pleasant to have teachers whom we and our friends knew. To find Dr. Cheever and Dr. Bremer so cordial and agreeable in the School and then to meet them again in the Somerset Ballroom engendered a sort of kindred spirit. These men were important in the School, and now we belonged also. They treated us considerately and tried earnestly to help us, and we in turn were encouraged to live up to their expectations. The atmosphere was friendly and it was stimulating.

On Monday, October 19, dissection of the human body was begun. Ours was a good table: George and I worked on the arm, Bill Reggio, George's college roommate, and Harry Lyman on the leg, and Don Knowlton and Phil Wilson on the head. On the second night this table dined together in the homey grillroom, with its open fire, in the basement of the Hotel Victoria — it is now a flower shop — and then rolled out, six of us in the same cab, to the first social meeting of H.M.S. Class of 1912.

On Wednesday, October 21, we had our first quiz. I remember it well, for this particular quiz was a turning point in my own personal education. Dr. Elisha Flagg, instructor for our table, was a big, tall man with a deep voice, very genial and pleasant, who took his duties lightly. When I hesitated over the answer to a fairly simple question, it was not Dr. Flagg, but my fellow students, George Minot in particular, who turned to me with a look that seemed to say: "What? You don't know *that?*" My chagrin was very real.

That first quiz showed more than anything else that times had changed. Today on the mantelpiece of Dean Hanford's house in Cambridge — he was Dean of Harvard College under President Lowell — is a photograph of an etching of President Lowell, inscribed in these words over the signature: "Dean A. Chester Hanford, In gratitude to his fellow-laborer in raising the respect for scholarship in Harvard College."

In the college of our time scholarship did not command respect. On the contrary, if a man received all A's and B's in his courses, it was assumed that there was something a little queer about him. This may have accounted for George's reticence about his senior grades at Harvard. In the Medical School, the attitude was quite different. George continued to get A's in all his courses. He knew more than any of us, and his knowledge gave him satisfaction. The respect that each one of us had for him developed at that first quiz, and increased as our lives went on.

On Saturday, December 26, George and I went to "Chappy." It was a wonderful day, almost like summer. I went in swimming for a quick dip; the water was too cold for George. Each day we tramped over the island, taking a lunch with us. We came back to town a week later, each like a new man.

In the second term, Dr. Walter B. Cannon gave his course in physiology in the mornings, and we studied biochemistry in the afternoons. In physiology, we worked with frogs, guinea pigs, and cats. My notes of Dr. Cannon's lectures say nothing directly about the study of digestion by x-ray, and yet he had been working on the problem since 1898. Evidently he was not ready to tell us that the outlines of the stomach and the intestines can be revealed by adding bismuth to the test meal to make its progress visible by the x-ray. The gastrointestinal x-rays that are taken today, every day, in every hospital in the world, depend on Dr. Cannon's work.[1]

We made observations on body temperature and its regulation. It is interesting to see how close Dr. Cannon came in 1909 to understanding the principles of the basal metabolism. Although Friedrich Mueller, back in 1893, had suspected that patients with thyrotoxicosis from too much thyroid hormone used up food at a rate faster than normal, it was not until several years after we had graduated that Francis G. Benedict, Graham Lusk, Eugene F. Dubois, and our friend James H. Means made practical use of measurements of the basal metabolism.

In the afternoons of that term, Dr. Otto Folin and our college teacher, Dr. Lawrence J. Henderson, instructed us in biological chemistry. Dr. Henderson was much interested in the equilibrium between acids and bases in physiological systems. It was Dr. Henderson who recognized that the concentration of hydrogen ions is proportional to the ratio between the concentration of carbonic acid ions and the concentration of bicarbonate ions. At the time of his lectures to us, he was writing his monograph[2] on the subject. In later years, the investigations of Dr. Henderson and his associates were to explain the many interrelations between the components of the blood: the ability of hemoglobin in the red blood cells to take up oxygen in the lungs and to release it in the tissues, and of the blood plasma to carry carbon dioxide from the tissues to the lungs and at the same time to maintain the pH at its proper neutral level. He demonstrated in quantitative terms how well the blood fulfills its complex functions.

Now, in our second semester, we were not confused by Dr. Henderson's discussion of the electrolytes and their dissociation. We could follow his argument about salts, and we could comprehend what he told us about hemoglobin. We could understand the mass law, which says: "The effect of a substance in a chemical reaction is proportional to its concentration." This last seemed easy enough — it was almost self-evident — and then one day Dr. Henderson began to talk about the "constant *K*." Dr. Henderson understood it, evidently, but I am not sure that even George knew what the "constant *K*" really was. I am sure that I never did.

Dr. Otto Folin, a delightful gentleman with a keen sense of humor in spite of a facial paralysis of long standing, was easier to understand. Carbohydrates, proteins, and fats were described in his lectures and illustrated in his laboratory. It was Dr. Folin who was soon to describe[3] a number of simple methods for several chemical measurements that today are applied to almost every patient in almost every hospital. The determinations of the amounts of nonprotein nitrogen, uric acid, and sugar in the blood are made by procedures that were devised in their first form by Dr. Folin. His methods make use of visual color comparisons of unknown specimens against known standards. Today photoelectric colorimeters make the determinations quickly and accurately. Just think what the techniques of quantitative measurement introduced by Dr. Folin have accomplished!

In February, Dr. Maurice H. Richardson, Moseley Professor of of Surgery, invited a number of us to dine at his house. He was *the* surgeon of Boston, a highly successful practitioner and a very skillful operator, who took excellent care of all his patients. He was a big, fat man, slightly short of breath, dressed immaculately in a smooth dark-blue suit. His clean white shirt had a low collar and he wore a tie of plain color, often red, made into a large knot. He was jovial and talkative, and he seemed to enjoy us students. We had an interesting time that night, hearing him talk about his surgical experiences.

On a Sunday in February, several classmates came out to my father's house in Readville for luncheon, and we climbed Blue Hill in the afternoon. On Monday, Washington's birthday, George and I walked over Bear Hill and had our lunch on the edge of Ponkapoag Pond. Before we got home we had covered about ten miles.

On the long week end of May 30, the *Dorel* was under way for the first time. That summer in July, Bob Amory, Ned Wigglesworth, and I were with George on the cruise of the Eastern Yacht Club. The older men, in their larger ships, were very kind to us, and even more so when our crew won the rowboat race. That notoriety helped us. George stayed on the *Dorel* most of that summer.

In September 1909, my father bought an automobile. He sent me to Springfield, Massachusetts, to stay for a few days and to observe the assembly of a car in the Knox factory. It was a wise move, for those early cars were not too reliable. If the driver could recognize a loose wire or see that the float in the carburetor was stuck, he could make the thing go again. A little later I was to teach George to run the machine. He never did understand the mechanism and was never interested in it. Engines were man-made, and their physiology was much too mechanical.

On Thursday, September 30, 1909, our second year began. In the mornings we studied pathology under Dr. William T. Councilman, a thickset, stoutish man in his fifties, with wisps of brown hair trying to cover his bald head. He had come to Harvard from Johns Hopkins, where he had been associated with Dr. Welch and Dr. Osler, and he brought some of the Hopkins atmosphere with him. His work was slow and deliberate — and effective. He gave us time to study a few slides carefully instead of trying to race through the whole collection. He wanted our work to be thorough and accurate. He was an excellent teacher, but I doubt if we students appreciated that he was an expert on malaria or that he exerted an important influence on American medicine. Dr. Councilman had a somewhat hesitating speech; he talked in a low voice about the "cap-Hill-aries," with accent on the "hill," rather than on the "cap," and that amused us.

We spent long hours that fall looking through our microscopes and making drawings of what we saw. George's notebook constitutes almost a short textbook of pathology. For a man whose handwriting was almost illegible at times, and who had very little idea of artistic design, his drawings are surprisingly good. He was meticulous about recording what he saw as accurately as possible, and, being inquisitive by nature, he tried to show details as well as the general picture.

Bacteriology as we know it today was in its infancy in 1909. Dr. Harold C. Ernst tried hard to teach us what the different organisms looked like and how they could be distinguished one from the other. His bacteriology was like botany — a study of forms and of classifications. Little was then known about the actions of bacteria — the ways in which they produced disease or the reasons why certain individuals were resistant to their invasion while others were not. It was not until some years later that Dr. Hans Zinsser was called from New York to be Professor of Bacteriology and Immunology at Harvard Medical School, where he was the first to teach the students about immunology. George did not have him as a teacher, but he did have Dr. Zinsser as a friend who taught him vicariously and stimulated him.

George Minot's method of study was always logical and systematic. He could make beautiful summaries, with the material neatly arranged under A, B, and C, and then each section subivided under 1, 2, and 3. When quizzes or examinations came around, these summaries, each compressed onto one or two pages, were quite enough to emphasize the essentials and to help to recall the smaller details as well. His mind always worked in a clear, logical fashion, and no point was put down that was not quite clear in his own mind. If he did not know, he would ask the professor, or else look it up. Needless to say, his example helped me immensely.

On Wednesday, October 6, 1909, Mr. A. Lawrence Lowell was inaugurated as President of Harvard University. We young men went over to see the ceremony. As George had prophesied, it was a very impressive occasion. We joined the academic procession with pleasure and some awe, and listened to the speeches with real interest. For the moment, the new regime did not affect the mode of instruction then current at the Medical School.

At the beginning of the year, a small compliment was paid to George and me. Dr. David Cheever appointed us prosectors in anatomy. To demonstrate the muscles, the blood vessels, and the nerves, the specimen must be prepared beforehand, and this preparation gave last year's students a chance to review their anatomy. The task added something to our burdens, however, for on several evenings each week one or several of us would have to work in the dissecting room. As I look back on this experience, I marvel at the knowledge and skill of the modern surgeon who is able to identify the nerves and muscles without the slightest difficulty, while we students, with ample time and a bloodless field, had trouble in finding all that was required. Prosecting all alone in the bottom of a big building at midnight, with several dead bodies lying around on as many slab tables, was not the most pleasant of occupations.

In the second half of the second year, clinical teaching began, and we were introduced to patients for the first time. In the morning we were sent in sections to clinics at different hospitals, where we learned to take histories and to make examinations under the close supervision of an instructor. Our particular section was indeed fortunate, for we had a remarkable teacher. Our first meeting with Dr. George S. C. Badger stands out vividly. About fifteen of us were assembled in a room opposite the Female Medical Clinic in the Massachusetts General Hospital Outpatient Department. Dr. Badger came in, and we stood up. Then he left again without saying anything. We all sat down and went on with our chattering. The next time he came in, he brought a woman and seated her in a chair opposite us. Once more he disappeared, this time leaving the woman but saying nothing. We resumed our chatter but subdued it a little. When Dr. Badger came back for a third time he pointed quickly to one of us.

"What have you been observing about this woman?" No answer, of course.

"Next man! Was she limping when she came in?" No answer.

"Can she move her arms and all her fingers?" No answer.

"Is her breathing natural? What about her color? What about her general attitude? Is she suffering? Is she happy?"

Dr. Badger looked from one of us to the next, and when there was no response, he seemed disappointed. He was silent for a moment and then he turned on us.

"Gentlemen, you must never waste time; it is far too valuable. You must learn to be inquisitive and learn how to use your eyes. There is a good deal to be told about this woman just by looking at her. First of all, she is very thin. She does not look well. She did limp when she came in, and now notice her hands — the fingers are deformed and out of their normal position. She has arthritis in a severe form, but that is not the point. I asked her to sit in front of you because I hoped that, even without my prompting, you would see things about her that were, at the least, not normal. I wanted to impress on you the importance of observation. At all times, in all places, and under all circumstances, the doctor must look. Then, of course, he must try to *see* what he is looking at; and that last is the essence of education."

Many times I have thought what a wonderful way that was to begin our instruction: to drive home immediately the importance of direct observation. To this day, I am indebted to Dr. Badger.

In the second term of the second year a small group of us enjoyed a private extracurricular course given by Dr. Frederick T. Lord one evening a week at his house at 305 Beacon Street. This course was a review of Osler's textbook.[4] Each week several chapters were assigned, and we were to learn their contents and be ready to answer questions about them. This was teaching of the old-fashioned variety. To be sure, there was some chance to discuss Dr. Osler's findings and conclusions, but on the whole we were expected to "learn it cold" as we read it. This course with Dr. Lord forced us to read Osler, and read him carefully, and that in turn made our didactic lectures much more understandable, or conversely, if the lectures happened to come first, the reading was easier. A colossal amount of information — of cold, hard facts — was accumulated in those days.

During the summer after our second year (1910), it was advisable to "get rid of" the practical work in obstetrics if possible. George and I both had our services then, he at the Boston Lying-In Hospital on McLean Street, not far from the Massachusetts General Hospital, and I at the "Branch" over on Harrison Avenue in the South End of Boston. Dr. Howard T. Swain had given us a few talks on obstetrics during the spring, but our real instruction came from our own classmates. Each service lasted four weeks, in the first two of which we were assistants to the man just ahead. The technique, and most of the equipment, were handed down from one of us to the next in line.

One of our classmates tells of the accouchement on Merrimac Street, "third floor back." The Polish woman was having a rather hard time; the baby was coming slowly. As the medical student sat by her bedside, he happened to look over his shoulder. There was the husband, standing in the doorway with a gun over his arm.

"You get that baby and be quick about it," he said.

It was indeed fortunate that a few minutes later the uterine contractions became stronger, and the baby was born!

Obstetrics in midsummer in the slum districts was not always a pleasant experience, but it was usually safer than this. If we did walk through the "hole in the wall," a dark, filthy passage between Chambers Street and Leverett Street, behind the Massachusetts General, at three in the morning, we were not molested. Our doctor's bag seemed to protect us.

It was hot that summer. Cousin Jim had built a sort of glorified tent under the trees below his house in Milton. A wooden platform about ten by fifteen feet was big enough for four beds. The wooden frame over it held the canvas roof firmly in place, and the sides were covered with mosquito netting, as well as with khaki curtains that could be raised and lowered in case of wind or rain. It was delightful to sleep out of doors, where the air was sweet and the breeze was cool, and where in the morning the birds were right beside us. The idea came originally from Dr. Edward Livingston Trudeau, for whom Cousin Jim had great respect and admiration. When Dr. Trudeau founded the sanitarium at Saranac Lake, New York, he insisted that his patients be out of doors as much as possible, even in the middle of winter. Each of his cottages had a sleeping porch attached. Cousin Jim continued the idea when he made the children at the Prendergast Preventorium, which he founded, sleep in a sort of open tent, really a shed.

For a month in the summers of his second and third years at medical school, George was invited to help with the routine work of the Harvard Clinic, which was an interesting experiment. In 1909 the Faculty, under Dean Henry A. Christian, suggested that an outpatient clinic be established in the Medical School buildings, partly to give medical service to people in the neighborhood and to employees and partly to provide material for clinical teaching. In 1910 the Harvard Corporation approved the plan, and the clinic was started. George worked for several weeks under the visiting men — Doctors Francis W. Palfrey, George C. Shattuck, and Channing Frothingham, Jr. — and he enjoyed it.

Our third year started in the fall of 1910. Large teaching clinics were held every morning in one or another of the hospitals. The whole class attended and listened to the Chief of the medical or surgical staff, who was also the Professor of Medicine or Surgery, present one or two patients and explain their problems to us. The patient would sometimes walk in and sit in a chair in the amphitheater, but more often nurses and orderlies would push in the bed with the patient in it. What patient was chosen depended partly on the special interests of the instructor, partly on what cases were at hand. We liked these clinics, and enjoyed comparing the appearance of the patient and the history of his case with the description of the disease as it had been given us in lectures and textbooks. Whenever the patient showed variations from the regular patterns, the demonstration became even more interesting.

After the morning clinic, the class dispersed to its section assignments, sometimes in the outpatient department of the same hospital but often across town in a different hospital. Section work in medicine, surgery, diseases of the nose and throat, neurology, and eye disease came in rotation, and the assignments to them were usually for a month, sometimes for two.

Each afternoon we had to listen to three or four one-hour lectures from 2 P.M. until 6 P.M. It is hard to say how we stood that strain, and as for the lecturers who started their talks at 4 P.M., or, worse still, at 5 P.M., they must have had a difficult task to hold our attention. The lectures of Dr. Henry A. Christian were probably the best and most interesting. Dr. Christian talked in a deliberate manner, choosing his words carefully so that his secretary, who was hiding in the corner, could take down every word. At our twenty-fifth anniversary in 1937, he talked to us again and said: "During the lecture on nephritis, which I gave to you gentlemen on April 14, 1911, I asked Mr. Minot a question about treatment. I would like to know how Dr. Minot would answer the same question today."

"Well, Dr. Christian," George said, "I presume that in 1911 my answer was concerned only with drugs. Today we know that disorders of the kidney function have profound effects upon the total body chemistry — upon the relations among salts, protein waste products, and water — and the modern treatment attempts to correct the disturbances of those physicochemical relations."

In his lectures, Dr. Christian covered almost the whole field of medicine, giving us the important points much as one might read them in a good textbook. Some years later, the Curriculum Committee came to recognize that most of the systematic lectures of this sort could be omitted. If the students read their textbooks carefully lectures become unnecessary. The teaching clinics give sufficient opportunity to discuss the textbook description. Today the staffs of almost every hospital of any size give "Grand Rounds" once in every week or two. The purpose is to show and discuss before the whole staff patients who present some unusual or striking feature of their disease, or to present a difficult problem that needs the thought and advice of everybody. Needless to say, Grand Rounds are very instructive to all the doctors, students, and nurses who attend them.

On one morning during his third year at medical school, George took time out to attend one of the last rounds his father made as visiting physician to the Massachusetts General Hospital. There was a woman on the ward whose disease had been diagnosed as pernicious anemia. In a recent lecture, Dr. Christian had described briefly a disease then little known, called chronic family hemolytic (acholuric) jaundice.

The patient (M.G.H. Case Record E.M. 177079) was a woman of thirty-four who had been admitted for the third time that July. She had been in the hospital twice before with a disease unknown to both visiting physicians and house pupils. All her life she had been weak and debilitated, and had had a peculiar color. She had been aware of a large mass in her abdomen, which was her enlarged spleen. Back home in Göteborg, Sweden, she had been treated for anemia, but her pale color had persisted. Her hemoglobin was only 35 percent of normal and her red blood count was around 2 million cells per cubic millimeter, instead of the normal count of 5 million. On her two previous hospital admissions, the doctors had not been really satisfied with their conclusions about her, for the symptoms did not quite fit the diagnosis of pernicious anemia.

On that morning George Minot, third-year medical student, made the diagnosis of family jaundice in this woman. He remembered from Dr. Christian's lecture that in this disease, which simulates pernicious anemia in so many ways, the red blood cells are peculiar in that they will disintegrate when exposed to concentrations of salt in water which are lower than the optimal but not so low as to be injurious to the cells of normal people.

He asked for a sample of her blood, and in the laboratory he demonstrated the "increased fragility" of the red blood cells, which confirmed the diagnosis of chronic family jaundice. Later he showed that the woman's sister, who also had been considered to have pernicious anemia, had family jaundice, too.

Dr. Hugo O. Peterson of Worcester, Massachusetts, who was "Sub-Pup" on Cousin Jim's service, remembers the incident to this day and recalls the pleasant admiration for the young student which this remarkable diagnosis engendered among all the house officers. Dr. Peterson claims a little credit for encouraging George to go ahead with his researches in blood.

Pharmacology, which we studied that year, was given by Dr. Franz Pfaff, a stout, thickset German with a white goatee. He talked with a marked accent. A frog was injected on the table before us with various drugs, and the reaction of "zees fraugh" was noted. Since the outcome was always "paralazees of respiratzione und circulatzione," and it was only a question of time until the frog died, the demonstrations did not teach us much.

In a course in comparative pathology, George, with Channing Frothingham, Jr., who was a young instructor, made two investigations which were good enough to be published in medical journals. The subjects were new, and the work was done thoroughly. The first[5] was very simple research; it consisted in taking the temperature of normal rabbits twice a day for five days. The second[6] was concerned with the effect of the injection of heated beef bile into rabbits to see if degenerative changes in the arteries could be produced, but nothing showed.

In the clinical subjects, like surgery, orthopedics, obstetrics, and neurology, distinguished practitioners lectured to us, each course being a systematic survey of the field — a duplication of what one could find in any good textbook.

It was a privilege to have Dr. Theobald Smith himself talk to us about immunity. He was obviously an important person, and we found later that he was the discoverer of the great principle that disease can be transmitted by the bites of insects. He had found[7] that Texas fever in cattle was due to the bite of the cattle tick, which drew blood from one animal and injected it into another.

These lectures forced us to learn the systems of disease, and made us aware of the principal parts of each of these systems. It did help our reading — or, I should say, with good notes of good lectures, we did not need to read so much. Each lecturer stressed what to him seemed to be the important items, and no doubt this stress helped us more than we appreciated at the time. Today we know that the function of the good lecturer is merely to arrange the topics in their proper relation and to provide emphasis on important points, so that the student will know how to spend his time in the library with greater efficiency and a clearer objective.

There was one teacher whose method was different. Dr. Richard C. Cabot was a forceful man, with clear-cut ideas and a clear-cut way of expressing them, who gave us his exercises in case teaching. A case selected from his book would be assigned ahead of time, and at the weekly meeting of the whole class he would read the history to us and then ask questions. Dr. Cabot says in his introduction: "We [teachers] can present it [the case] precisely as it is met with in practice . . . then we can help the student to disentangle the essentials . . . By the students' answers and by their questions — which soon come thick and fast if encouraged — the teacher can find out the gaps in each student's knowledge." [8]

After the discussion, the "actual diagnosis of the case as it was proved by operation, by necropsy, or by the course of the symptoms" is revealed "with a buzz of interest," and this leads to further discussion in case the class was not close enough to the correct conclusion. Also, as Dr. Cabot says in his introduction; "the students must be called upon by *name*." He had the remarkable ability to remember the name of each of us; he never had to ask it twice, and he remembered us later on in our hospital work. Needless to say, he was an excellent teacher of both undergraduates and graduate students of medicine. His case-teaching exercises still go on, but today they deal with curent cases. They are published verbatim in the *New England Journal of Medicine* under the title "Case Records of the Massachusetts General Hospital — Weekly Clinicopathological Exercises Founded by Richard C. Cabot." As such, they are read and used for teaching and self-instruction by doctors all over the world.

Dr. Cabot is even better known as the founder of medical social service. It was he who pointed out that illness raises many problems: the need for special medicine and diets, the need for eyeglasses, false teeth, or artificial limbs, the need for convalescent care, the needs of relatives left unsupported — all these are often pressing, and the social worker may be of even greater help than the doctor. Dr. Cabot was fortunate to have Miss Ida B. Cannon, sister of Dr. Walter B. Cannon, to help him as the first head of the Social Service Department at the Massachusetts General Hospital. It was about this that George wrote his social ethics thesis in college.

After Christmas of our third year, Ned Wigglesworth, George, and I went to Chappaquiddick for five days, and this time we practiced a little medicine there. Captain Sandsbury showed us the hornlike callus that had developed on the rim of his right ear. Having just heard Dr. John Bowen lecture about cutaneous horns, we felt completely competent to deal with this one. A twenty-penny spike was put in the coal fire, and the Captain was asked to sit with his back to the stove, in a good light. "Don't worry," we said; "we shall try not to hurt you!" When all was ready, the spike, almost white-hot, was held in a pair of pliers and the point was applied directly to the Captain's ear. There was a puff of white smoke. The Captain groaned audibly, but he didn't move, and when it was over the horn was gone. Next day, his ear was "a leetle sore," he said, but he seemed almost as pleased as we were. What a tolerant gentleman he was!

In the second half of the third year, George took on an extra activity. Dr. Frederick T. Lord, our former quizmaster, had George and me appointed as part-time house officers for six months at the Channing Home, a small hospital not far from the Medical School. Dr. Lord was Visiting Physician to this forty-bed hospital, which was used for the active treatment of tuberculosis. There was laboratory work to be done, and occasional histories to be taken. We learned how to stain the specimens of sputum quickly and well, and George became interested to see whether the variations in the numbers of tubercle bacilli could be correlated with the patients' progress. He also had a chance to study the anemia that occurs in tuberculosis.

At the end of this third year came the examinations. From Thursday, June 1, to Wednesday, June 14, we passed through purgatory. We crammed for eleven examinations in as many working days. How we survived is hard to say. George's clear, orderly thinking and his remarkable memory, aided by his excellent notes, gave him honors in every subject, and I was helped by the example he had set me.

Later in June we were both called as "strikers" (substitute house pupils) to the Massachusetts General Hospital to help with laboratory work on the wards. Each day George and I drove in and out of town in my father's Hudson; my family were all at "Chappy" and I stayed with the Minots in Milton. Boston was hot again in the summer of 1911, and the tent out under the trees was appreciated greatly.

In late June and July, George worked in the Medical Outpatient Department at the Massachusetts General Hospital, taking histories and making physical examinations, improving his technique, and gaining more and more experience. In the afternoons, he went to the Harvard Clinic at the Medical School, where the pressure was less and the chance for more careful and thoughtful study of the patients was better.

While George was busy in the clinics, the *Dorel* was used at the beginning of that summer by George's brothers, Jimmy and Henry, who went off with their friends on several very successful cruises. Cousin Jim liked sailing well enough, but he did not care for the life on a small boat with four men sleeping in one cabin. Often, however, the boys would meet him at Bar Harbor and take him out for the day. In August, George spent his vacation cruising on the *Dorel,* and on September 1 I joined the ship at Bar Harbor. Orville Rogers, our classmate, was on board, and we had a wonderful two weeks on another cruise east into Passamaquoddy Bay.

Our fourth year was quite different from the previous years at the Medical School. Each month was devoted to a separate subject, on which we could work intensively. Medicine, surgery, and pathology were required, at least two months for each. The other courses, like laryngology, dermatology, and ophthalmology, which took only one month, were optional. During this year our routine was much less exacting; we had a little time to think. Also we had some time to play. Several times in the fall George and I went to the country, either for golf or for a good hike through the Blue Hills Reservation. After Thanksgiving, we spent the week end at the Seapuit Club in Osterville on Cape Cod, where the oysters were obtained right out of the bay in front, and where the golf course was open all winter.

One highlight of our fourth year was the course in surgery with Dr. Maurice H. Richardson, the Moseley Professor, who had invited some of us to dinner three years before. The course consisted in following Dr. Richardson on his rounds for just one whole day. The men in our section took turns, two at a time. At 8 A.M. Dr. Richardson's house at 224 Beacon Street was a busy place. Downstairs in the offices were the nurses and the assistant, Dr. Richard H. Miller, hustling to assemble as many kits of instruments as there were operations scheduled. Upstairs were Mrs. Richardson and her younger boys, finishing breakfast. Mrs. Richardson called us up for extra coffee and another piece of toast: "You'd better eat now while you can, for you won't get any lunch today." In a few minutes the doctor began to bellow from the front door, "Hurry up. It's time to go. Get a move on!"

Outside stood two open Pierce Arrows, with the brass all shiny. Dr. Richardson climbed onto the front seat of the first car, beside the chauffeur. George and I had the whole tonneau to ourselves. In the doctor's hand was a large rubber bulb, which he could squeeze to produce a deep moan. As he squeezed it at almost every crossroad, there was no doubt that we were coming. Behind us was the second car, driven by Dr. Miller, with the nurses and the bags containing the instruments.

On arrival at the Corey Hill Hospital the team went straight to their positions, the two nurses going to the operating room, where the instruments were put to boil while they were scrubbing. Dr. Miller went up to do several dressings before he went to the operating room. Dr. Richardson was not in such a hurry. He saw his patient and told him not to worry but to "just do what they tell you," and then he talked with the patient's friends to assure them that the operation would be easy and successful. After that he said good morning to several older patients; and as he had an extra minute, he played a tune on the piano in the hall. When he reached the operating room, all was ready.

Dr. Richardson took pride in two things: the speed with which he could remove the appendix, and the smallness of the incision that he required. His dexterity was remarkable.

When the operation was over, the instruments were gathered up, the nurses put on their overcoats, and we sped from the Corey Hill over to the Baptist Hospital, and then later to the Vincent Hospital. In each place the procedure was quite the same; the members of the team had been trained well.

In the middle of the morning a message came for Dr. Richardson, and we heard him say, "Tell her we'll be there at about twelve o'clock."

When the operation was finished, he turned to us: "Come on, boys, get your coats. We're off to Weston. Dr. Van Nuys has a patient who he thinks has appendicitis." We went out fast, quite as if we were going to a fire, the horn moaning frequently. On our arrival, however, the haste vanished.

Looking back now, I can see Dr. Richardson sitting in the parlor, hearing the story from the patient's attractive young wife, while we students fidgeted in the background. He gave her the impression that he had nothing to do for the rest of the day except to look after her husband. Upstairs, his examination was thorough; and as he sat on the side of the bed, his whole attitude radiated confidence and assurance. "I am sorry that you have this trouble," he said, "but there is no doubt about the cause of it, and I can tell you that the treatment is easy and you need not worry about it. Your appendix will come out this afternoon. Your wife will take you to the hospital and I shall meet you there at about four o'clock. We shall fix it for you; you will be all right." No questions were asked; the need for operation was assumed. There was no alternative. There was no need to bother about arrangements; they were quite unnecessary. Dr. Richardson would take care of everything. His sincerity, his kindliness, and his consideration for the patient and his family produced a confidence that left no room for doubt or argument.

The visit took less than half an hour, and after it back we sped to town. Dr. Richardson's house was quiet this time. A few patients were in the waiting room, Dr. Richardson disappeared into the inner office, and we students went upstairs, where Mrs. Richardson gave us crackers and cheese, doughnuts and milk. At about 3:30 P.M. we were off again, to operate on the patient from Weston promptly and efficiently, as promised.

Whenever the car was moving, Dr. Richardson would turn around and talk to us about the patient we had just seen, and about other cases, too. He had the faculty of sharing his enthusiasm, as well as his knowledge, with us. He liked to teach, probably because he liked people. He was a real Doctor — with a capital "D."

The course in fourth-year medicine was divided then, as it is now, into sections that met in the different hospitals. At the Massachusetts General Hospital, the course in medicine was given by Dr. Francis W. Palfrey. Each morning the six or eight of us in the section would assemble in the Pathology Laboratory, where Dr. Palfrey would lead the discussion about the patients whom we had studied the day before. The student would read his history of the case and describe his physical findings, and then outline the treatment that he would advise. Then we would go up to the ward and gather around the bed. Dr. Palfrey was a quiet little man, very serious, but he was an excellent practitioner. He would examine the patient most carefully, and then he would ask questions. Were the little red spots part of the venous or the arterial systems and how could we tell? Was the noise to be heard in the chest râles due to mucus in the bronchial tubes or was it a friction rub due to pleurisy? If it was pleurisy, would the rub develop in a few hours; if so, what was the disease? Was the diagnosis more likely to be tuberculosis or was it pneumonia?

The treatment that the student advised was compared with the actual orders written in the order book, and thus the reasons for prescribing the various drugs were discussed and compared with their known pharmacological actions. I remember Dr. Palfrey's remark: "The nursing care on this ward is excellent. How do you know that the patient would not have improved anyway, whether or not he was given drugs?" Dr. Palfrey taught us to be critical.

In those days, we students wrote out our histories and "physicals," but our writing was never incorporated into the official record. Occasionally a house pupil (or intern, as they are called today) would fall sick, and then the best fourth-year student would be called in to "strike" on the service. During that time, the histories and the examinations that he described were official.

Today all this is different. The fourth-year students have become "clinical clerks." The histories that they take on the new cases are excellent. The students make physical examinations, too, and now their work is incorporated into the record — subject, of course, to review and correction by the house officer. In doing this, the student of today has the sense of responsibility and importance that in our day was not felt, and in consequence his work is much better, and incidentally the burden on the house staff is reduced considerably.

On April 1, our month in a special course in pathology with Dr. J. Homer Wright began. Dr. Wright had a gruff exterior, but inside he was very human. One morning George had an interesting slide. He asked Dr. Wright if he would look at it. Dr. Wright, engrossed in his own work, pretended not to hear George's plea. Finally, however, he slowly looked up from his microscope with obvious annoyance, turned, and said just two words: "Oh — Hell." In a moment, however, the presence of George Minot seemed to penetrate his consciousness, and he added, "What have you got there?" After that, all was well, and Dr. Wright launched into his explanation of the blood platelets.

In 1906, Dr. Wright had discovered that the large cells of the bone marrow — the giant cells known as megakaryocytes — had a very irregular outline from which fragments became detached, and he believed that these fragments became the blood platelets that are concerned with the clotting process.[9] Dr. Wright was doing important work on the blood, and this work appealed to George. Incidentally, it was Dr. Wright who discovered a good stain for routine blood smears, and "Wright's stain" is still used today in many hospital laboratories. It was fortunate that George knew how to make friends with Dr. Wright, for, once inside the austere, almost unapproachable, shy demeanor, he found a wealth of interesting information, and in the finding he absorbed some of Dr. Wright's enthusiasm.

When we look back at the course of study through which we passed, and at the eminent men who directed it, it is not surprising that graduates of the Harvard Medical School did well in their life work. I believe, however, that the H.M.S. Class of 1912 was outstanding. We graduated fifty-five men. Besides George Minot, Nobel prize winner, the class includes five heads of university medical school departments, a member of the Rockefeller Foundation, and a president of the American Medical Association.

4

Massachusetts General Hospital

In our fourth year at the Medical School, we all began to think about what was coming next. At graduation, in June 1912, the degree of Doctor of Medicine awarded to us would imply that we were qualified to go out on our own and practice our new profession. One or two of our classmates did just that. One, for example, bought himself a microscope and some other simple equipment, and left for Nebraska, from where he wrote later on that his microscope was the only one in that section of the country. Subsequently that man did extremely well, and was beloved by the countless patients who came to him.

Most of the class, however, were made aware of the great difference between the theory and the practice of physic. To obtain an internship in a large teaching hospital meant that the mass of facts that had been learned from books, lectures, and clinics could be applied in the beginning under competent supervision. We had training, but we needed experience.

George Minot wanted to obtain this experience at the Massachusetts General Hospital if possible. His reason for this was that he had been brought up in the M.G.H. tradition. The Massachusetts General Hospital was an old, highly respected institution of Boston. Our families and friends had been closely concerned with its work and its support. The Visiting Physicians and Surgeons were outstanding doctors and excellent teachers. George's father and my grandfather had each contributed his knowledge and wisdom to the Hospital. It is true that George had been watching the construction of the Peter Bent Brigham Hospital with interest, but it would not be ready for another year.

On Wednesday, January 17, 1912, George and I, with several

others, took our examinations for Medical "House Pupil" * at the Massachusetts General Hospital. Our trials were held in the office of Dr. Herman F. Vickery, one of the Visiting Physicians, who lived at 263 Beacon Street. It is an interesting coincidence that my family live today in that same house. The room in which we were examined in 1912 is the very room in which I practice medicine today, and in which I am writing this account.

About twelve of us, who had the courage to hope that we might be among the six chosen, assembled there that evening. We sat upstairs in the dining room — tense, anxious, and speechless — and then one by one we were called downstairs to Dr. Vickery's office and to our fate. It was not a pleasant experience. Dr. Vickery's office was a fair-sized room. The members of the examining board — Dr. Vickery, Dr. Frederick C. Shattuck, Dr. James J. Minot, and Dr. Elbridge G. Cutler — were sitting around the fire, smoking their cigars. The victim was directed to the empty chair that stood by the corner of the mantelpiece. In the middle of the room there was a low table with cigars and cigarettes on it. We wondered later whether the temptation to smoke had been a trap to test our manners, but fortunately none of us had helped himself. To this day I remember the first question: "What are the causes of coma?" and the second: "What subject in medicine interests you most?" It was quite an ordeal, but George R. Minot, Orville F. Rogers, John E. Talbot, Oswald H. Robertson, John W. Hammond, and I passed it.

On the ninth of July, many of our class from the Harvard Medical School went to the State House in Boston to take the examinations given by the State Board of Registration in Medicine. It was a nuisance, of course, but failure to pass carried possibilities of trouble quite enough to make us worry about it a little. We passed safely, and became full-fledged physicians, licensed to practice medicine in Massachusetts. Though we were now qualified accord-

* Mrs. Grace Whitney Myers tells us that the term "House Pupil" was adopted in 1849 in place of the terms "House Physician" and "House Surgeon." This was on account of the early practice of choosing assistants from among *students* of medicine in the last year of their course of study instead of the later practice of selecting *doctors* of medicine who had just received their diplomas. In February 1922, the term "House Pupil" was officially changed to "House Officer." ("House Pupil," "House Officer," and "Intern" all mean the same thing.) Grace Whitney Myers, *History of the Massachusetts General Hospital June, 1872, to December, 1900* (Boston, 1929), p. 31.

ing to the law, according to our own estimation we had only begun to learn.

George's service at the hospital began officially on August 1, but every house pupil was asked to appear two weeks ahead of the starting date, so as to allow time for vacations later on. In early July, George and I took another ride in my father's Hudson, which I tried to teach George to run. He got his automobile driver's license in August.

The Massachusetts General Hospital is located in the West End of Boston, a good mile along the Charles River from the Minot house at 188 Marlborough Street. The first hospital building, which opened for patients in September 1821, was designed by Charles Bulfinch and was situated on the shore of the Charles River. It provided four wards, each with about twenty-five beds. There is an interesting old print that shows a patient being landed from a sailboat at the hospital wharf. Wings were added to the Bulfinch Building in 1846, built of the granite "hammered and fitted for use by the convicts at Charlestown," as Dr. Joseph Garland quoted it in his scholarly review,[1] and this Bulfinch Building serves in pictures as the symbol of the entire hospital. In our day, the four medical wards were in the east end of the Bulfinch Building and the four surgical wards in its west end. Each ward held about twenty-eight beds, and each was a large, almost square, room, with a big chimney in the center and fireplaces in the front and back of it. On cold bleak days in winter, the open fire was cheerful and comfortable, but it was not often lit. When the Bulfinch was made fireproof in 1934, the chimney was removed; comfort gave way to efficiency.

In the center of the Bulfinch was a dome with a glass section that lighted the amphitheater under it. This "ether dome" was the room in which the inhalation of sulfuric ether as an anesthetic agent was first demonstrated by Dr. William Thomas Green Morton, a Boston dentist, on October 16, 1846. On that day, the surgeon, Dr. John Collins Warren, removed a tumor from the jaw of his patient. When the patient declared that he had felt no pain during the operation, Dr. Warren turned to the distinguished company and said, "Gentlemen, this is no humbug." The Bulfinch Building, with its Ether Dome, is almost a shrine to those who have worked at the M.G.H.

The main entrance to the hospital was at the east end of the Bulfinch Building. Here were the offices of the Superintendent and his assistants, as well as the offices of the Nurses' Training School. There was a small information desk with a telephone switchboard behind it. Patients were brought to the hospital by horse and carriage, including an M.G.H. horse ambulance driven by Tom Lee, the hackdriver. On arrival they were carried on a stretcher to the wards upstairs, or else wheeled on a stretcher-truck to the Accident Room, which was in the north end of the old Bigelow Building.

It is hard to realize that until the Phillips House was erected in 1917, there were no private patients in the Massachusetts General Hospital. It is true that we had Jackson Ward B, a temporary structure with eight large rooms designed for special patients, but it was used mostly by the surgeons, and they were not supposed to charge for their services to the "private" patients in it.

For the treatment of patients, the facilities of the hospital as well as the doctors were divided into four services: the East and West Surgical Services and the East and West Medical Services. Each one had its own staff of visiting men, one of whom was Chief, and of course there were also the house pupils, whose services on either East or West were entirely comparable, except that the different visiting physicians might have different approaches to the problems of the patients. In the Bulfinch Building, all the wards on the second floor housed male patients, and all on the third floor housed female, so that each service had one ward on each floor.

On July 15, 1912, George Minot became "Sub-Pup" on the East Medical Service. Orville Rogers began on the West. The East and West Medical and Surgical Services each had four house pupils, who worked up through four positions — Sub-Pup, Pup, Junior, and Senior — holding each one for four months, to make a total of sixteen months. Every four months, each man moved up to a position of greater responsibility until, as Senior, he became for four months the doctor in charge of about sixty patients, subject, of course, to the advice of the visiting man.

The Medical Sub-Pup worked in the Out-Patient Department in the mornings, and helped on the wards — "In the House," we called it — in the afternoons. The Pup was in charge of all laboratory work in the House. When the Junior was out, the Pup covered for him, taking histories and making physical examinations. The Junior and Senior took care of the patients and were responsible for their welfare. The Senior House Pupil had real standing in the hospital.

George found the first two weeks of his service in the hospital strenuous. As Sub-Pup, he began his day at 8:30 A.M. in the Out-Patient Department. Here came a long line of "old" patients wanting a little more advice and the renewal of their prescriptions. Some needed further physical examinations to check previous findings and to follow the progress of their diseases. For the first time, George was free to advise treatment on his own responsibility and as he thought best. He could repeat the physical examinations in order to check on previous findings, and he could ask the patients to come again so that he could observe the changes in their condition and be ready to help them further. There were one or two assistant Visiting Physicians on duty in the Out-Patient Department for a few hours in the morning of each day, and there were a few medical students. The visiting men examined most of the new cases and started the treatment indicated, and the students helped them by taking histories. In those days, however, the students had no definite position in the routine. No one counted on them, but if they could help, so much the better.

It was the House Pupil who did most of the work and who took care of a large share of the patients who had been there before. Not many of the visiting men took the time to see again the patients whom they had originally seen as new cases.

If toward the end of the morning, when the Visiting Physician had gone home, there were new cases left, it was the House Pupil who took their histories, made tentative diagnoses, and began their treatment. It was usually late when he had finished. The dining room closed at two o'clock, and if he was too late for lunch there, he had to get along on the milk and crackers that the head nurse on the ward would give him.

The Medical Out-Patient Department in 1912 had two parts — the male clinic downstairs and the female upstairs — and the House Pupil spent two months in each. Each section had a large office and waiting room, a row of examining rooms, and a laboratory with facilities adequate for routine examinations of urine, blood, and sputum. How curious that this well-constructed fireproof building, erected in 1906, was not provided with electric lights! No one expected that it would be used at night, or even in the late afternoon.

Equally remarkable, there was no telephone in the Out-Patient Department for some years. If the call were really urgent, a messenger would come over from the Accident Room, and the visiting man would have to walk to the next building. The first telephone was not installed there until about 1919.

During the afternoons, the Sub-Pup helped with the laboratory work in "the House." In theory, the Pup was off duty every other afternoon and evening, and the Out-Patient man — the Sub-Pup — took over. In practice, however, there was no "off duty." There was so much to do that both men were busy most of the time. With a big clinic requiring intensive work in the morning, and with a long list of laboratory determinations to be made in the afternoon and evening, the day did not end until 10:30 or 11 P.M. No wonder George felt tired.

When George became Pup in December 1912, his life was quite different. He was in the House now, and he felt that he was a very real and not unimportant part of the Massachusetts General Hospital. This was what he had been waiting for.

The Pup was responsible for all laboratory studies on the ward patients. Each morning the bench in the laboratory was graced with a long row of urine glasses and a number of small china pots containing stools. After a few days he learned how to take specific gravities, how to line up wine glasses, put a small sample of urine and a few cubic centimeters of nitric acid into each to test for albumin, and how to put urine and Fehling's solution into test tubes, and then to let the tubes stand in boiling water to see if sugar were present. The urine sediments took more time. George's descriptions of the number of squamous cells and their character, the white cells, whether separate or in clumps, and even the debris, make interesting reading. For him, the ordinary routine was not enough. Fancy tests, such as those for acetone, diacetic acid, or bile, were made occasionally. Ehrlich's reagent for urinobilogen was applied quite often, but just what the result told us about the patient, or how it modified either diagnosis or treatment, was never very clear.

There was a quantitative test for urine sugar which was simple and interesting. Yeast will convert sugar into carbon dioxide gas and either acetic acid or alcohol, and the amount of sugar can be calculated simply by observing the drop in the specific gravity of the sample before and after incubation — and the only incubator was in Dr. J. Homer Wright's laboratory. One evening a House Pupil (the name is withheld) laid the quart bottle of urine with yeast added on its side with the stopper against the door of the incubator. When next morning Dr. Wright came to look at his cultures, he opened the door, the stopper popped out with the gas pressure behind it, and the urine went all over him. What Dr. Wright said can not be recorded here — possibly! How George Minot laughed whenever he told that story.

One of the Pup's duties was to plant a new broth culture of typhoid bacilli each night. If the patient has typhoid fever, the antibody in the blood serum will cause typhoid bacilli to agglutinate — to clump together — in the so-called Widal test. The technique was to place nine loopfuls, or drops, of living culture on a glass slide, add one loopful of blood serum, mix the ten drops together, and cover with a cover glass. If agglutination is present, the masses of clumped organisms are easy to see under the microscope, and the test is positive. How much of the typhoid culture was spilled on the desk, how much was spread by flies and other insects is not known. It is fortunate that we House Pupils had all had inoculations of typhoid vaccine. Over the years, only one man came down with typhoid fever.

Stools excited George's special interest, for they were the residue of food and their character was related to diet. His descriptions of them were complete, including the fat globules, the muscle fibers, and sometimes the blood cells which were to be seen under the microscope.

Between ten and eleven o'clock in the morning, the Ward Visit began. The Pup knew little about the patients, but since questions about his laboratory findings might come up, he was supposed to be present. In the afternoons, the Pup made counts and smears of the blood cells. My own service at the Hospital followed immediately after George's, and I still shudder as I think of the long list of such examinations that George assigned me on my first day. In medical school, to finish a white count and blood smear had been a fair assignment for one afternoon, and now we were asked to make ten or a dozen such counts "between now and midnight — or else!" I knew that George himself had been appalled at first by the long list of tests required. It did not take him long, however, to learn to do white counts and smears quickly and accurately.

In the afternoons, there were also special activities, such as chest taps or spinal punctures. In one case, George took almost a page to describe the pleural fluid from a patient with a liver abscess (M.G.H. Case Record E.M. 187058). It is a masterpiece of good observation. When the stain sudan III demonstrated fat, George extracted the specimen with ether so as to demonstrate and measure the fat residue when the ether had evaporated. The fat proved the connection between the pleura and the liver.

It was the blood that interested George most of all. The descriptions that he wrote as Pup are meticulous in their exactness. The other house pupils recognized his interest and began to ask him, "Please look at this section," and "What do you think of that?" Early in his career he became an authority on diseases of the blood.

In 1912 and 1913 neither the Sub-Pup nor the Pup lived in the Hospital. At first George and Orville Rogers lived with Cousin Jim. After breakfast, they would walk along the embankment of the Charles River, to begin work at 8:30. If it was a nice day, the walk to the Hospital was pleasant, but in the nighttime, after fifteen hours of intensive effort, the mile walk home at midnight was not quite so refreshing. When my service began on November 14, George, Orville, and I rented a suite in the Charlesbank Homes next door to the Hospital. It was Cousin Jim who saw the building and gave us the idea, and then arranged the details for us. The building was brand new and it was of fireproof construction, with concrete floors and solid walls. Each room could be cleaned with a hose if one wanted to clean that way. There was a gas stove in the kitchen, and there were two soapstone washtubs which we found ideal for ice and beer. We had a good shower bath. The rooms were small but adequate, and we were very comfortable. It was a good place to sleep in.

The Juniors and Seniors on the East and West Medical Services lived in the Hospital. The House Pupils' "Flat" was just over the Accident Room. A narrow flight of stairs led up to it. The sitting room was on the second floor and overlooked the lawn in front of the Bulfinch. There were a number of small bedrooms on this floor and on the one above. The sitting room became our home. It had a fireplace, and in the corner stood an icebox well stocked with milk, ginger ale, and beer. There were crackers and cheese in another corner. One of us was elected "purveyor," and it was his duty to collect small contributions with which to buy supplies.

The Flat had a piano, as well as drums and one or two large tin cracker boxes for cymbals. When Bill Reggio beat the drums and Lyman Barton played the piano, the music was pretty good, and when everybody sang, our worries about sick patients vanished temporarily.

There was no telephone on the wards, but the Flat had a sort of local house phone, with a set of bell buttons at the bottom of the stairs. By ringing the appropriate bell, the nurse could reach any one of us in the middle of the night. In the daytime or evening, when she wanted a doctor, she pushed the big button, which rang a much louder bell. Whenever this bell rang, all noise stopped instantly, and then the nurse would call plaintively, "Dr. Minot," or "Dr. Wilson." If he were there, the "callee" went downstairs to the "caller," but if the callee was not in the Flat, one of us started counting softly, "One, two, three," and at the "Go," everyone joined in a roaring "NO!"

Mollie — good old Mollie — had been taking care of M.G.H. house officers for years. She had rheumatic heart disease with mitral stenosis, and had trouble on the stairs, but she made our beds and kept our rooms clean and in some sort of order. She was devoted to us, and all of us were devoted to her.

The bathroom was on the third floor, over the living room. It was a fair-sized place, with four washbasins and three large tubs. In the morning, the water in all tubs was left running, so that they were always full. The end tubs had hot water; the middle one had cold. On getting up, most men would lie in the hot tub for a minute or so and then would jump directly into the cold tub, usually with a yell, and with the water splashing all over. Fortunately, the asphalt floor was watertight and sloped to a drain in the middle. Life was simple and intimate, and it was very pleasant; even fastidious George liked it.

The House Pupils ate in the Staff Dining Room, close to the main kitchen. The food varied; George Minot did not much care for calves' brains and tripe, but we did not really have them often. At midnight, the food served in a corner of the kitchen was much better. Here was Maggie, genial and devoted, who was always glad to see us.

"What'll ye be havin' this time, one egg or two?" Her brogue was as big as her heart.

"One egg will be enough, thank you, Maggie."

"Sure, and ye've been workin' hard; ye better have two!"

"Can I have a piece of that cake?"

"Sure thing ye can — and there's a raisin in this piece."

Our nourishment at midnight was more than a snack; it was a real meal, and we needed it, for we had been working hard all evening, and it was now about five hours since supper. We enjoyed our suppers in Maggie's kitchen — and all the more so since they were against the rules!

Dr. Frederic A. Washburn was Superintendent of the Hospital. An Army colonel with a typical military posture and attitude, he was a gruff, unapproachable person, and a strict disciplinarian. Most people were afraid of him. He was an excellent housekeeper — the hospital was immaculate at all times — and he was very careful about spending money. There were no luxuries, whether personal, medical, or scientific. It was he who took away the side pockets in our trousers; we learned to walk with our hands in the back pockets. (Dr. George H. Bigelow, who became Superintendent in February 1934, when Dr. Washburn resigned, replaced the pants pockets as one of his first reforms.)

Dr. Washburn made rules about our conduct, and the Reading of the Rules was a ceremony that had to be attended with every change of service by every one of us unless he were excused. The roll was called each time. Needless to say, we didn't like this. One day, all the House Pupils formed in lock step behind our clarinet player, and marched all the way up to and into the Ether Dome in step with martial music, played very softly. That settled it; the rules were never read again! We House Pupils might be young and frivolous at times, but after all we were a selected group, and each was the holder of two university degrees. We were children no longer.

We had a little sentiment about the service to which we belonged. To emphasize our team play, the East Medical Service wore at one time bow ties of gaudy colors, all just alike, much to the envy of the other services; it was George's idea.

As Junior Medical House Pupil, George took case histories. One need question neither their accuracy nor their completeness. Every phase of the patient's problem was investigated and described. George's personal interest in food, eating, and digestion came out in his talks with patients: "Where do you eat? Is it a pleasant place? How much time do you take? Do you have someone to talk to? Do you chew your food?" And then, "What do you usually have for breakfast — and for lunch, and for dinner?" The matter of diet was always a matter of primary concern to George. For patients with pernicious anemia particularly, George was fussy about the diet. Even in that early time, he had an idea that there might be a relation between the disease and the total food intake.

His orders for diets were careful: "Beef tea, tea, water, dry toast, soft eggs, milk, and butter." "Add toast, coffee, lean meat, rice, custard, beef broth, and albumin water." "Allow any food patient desires, and at any time." "Try to get her to take as much as possible, a little each time, liquids preferably." "Feed meat, eggs, albumin water." "Add butter, custard, and cocoa." There were no dietitians in our time.

When George was Junior, the Visiting Physician was Dr. Frederick T. Lord, the one who had given us, in our third year of medical school, the special extracurricular quizzes on Osler's textbook. Dr. Lord was a short, stocky little man, with a springy walk, and with a bright twinkle in his eye. He was a thorough student of medicine, who knew all the possibilities of differential diagnosis. His stethoscope was the same kind that we had, but he could use it with wonderful effectiveness. He could hear the slightest abnormal sound in the chest, and quite often when we had been a bit doubtful about his demonstration we would discover on the next day that, sure enough, the lesion — a patch of pneumonia, for example — had developed so that signs of it were obvious. Dr. Lord was not quite as interested in treatment as he was in diagnosis, but that was just as well because it gave us — George particularly — a good opportunity to observe the effects of the drugs and of the diet which we had planned and ordered with such care.

Later, during George's Senior Service (my Junior Service) Dr. David L. Edsall, the new Jackson Professor of Clinical Medicine, visited on the East Medical Service, and we realized at once that to make rounds with him was a great privilege. Up to 1912, neither the Hospital nor the Harvard Medical School had had experience with a full-time paid professor in the clinical departments, nor had they had the funds to support him. The treatment of patients in the Hospital, as well as the teaching of students, was left to the voluntary services of those distinguished practitioners who were willing to give a part of their time in return for the experience and the prestige that the honorary position gave them. The new policy, which would give the clinical professor a permanent position with a salary sufficient to let him devote most of his time to teaching and research, had been an advance of tremendous significance.

A precedent was broken when Dr. Edsall was appointed from outside Boston. The new order said that the Jackson Professor of Clinical Medicine, who would also be Chief of Medicine at the M.G.H., must be the best-qualified man obtainable from anywhere. The Massachusetts General Hospital and the Harvard Medical School must work together so closely that they would agree on one man who would be appointed to both positions.

When Dr. Shattuck retired in 1911 from the active staff of the Hospital, and resigned the Jackson Professorship in the Medical School, a great effort was made to find a new Chief of Medicine who knew how to develop research and clinical investigation. It was Dr. Edwin A. Locke who knew Dr. Edsall and who introduced him to the trustees.

Dr. David Linn Edsall had been Professor of Pharmacology and Therapeutics at the University of Pennsylvania, with its Ayer Clinical Laboratory, where he had done important work on various disorders of metabolism. More recently he had been Professor of Preventive Medicine at the Washington University Medical School in

Saint Louis, Missouri. He was large, both in body and soul, direct in his point of view, broad in his knowledge, and profound in his wisdom. He was at least six feet five inches tall, and from his big frame came a deep voice with a kindly, sincere expression in it. Everyone was impressed by Dr. Edsall. To all his house officers and students he was stimulating and helpful. He was an excellent teacher, and within a year or two he had established a new idea at the Hospital — the idea that a really careful study of the patient as a whole might lead to a better understanding of his symptoms and the mechanism of their production. To all of us, and especially to men with natural inquisitiveness like James H. Means, Paul D. White, and George R. Minot, he was an inspiring leader.

On August 1, 1913, George became Senior on the East Medical Service and was in charge of two wards with twenty-eight patients in each, and of varying numbers (one to eight, perhaps) of patients in single rooms in the lower wards. I was his Junior. The Visiting Physician would discuss the case, he might find some point that George had overlooked, he might change the emphasis on the various factors, but, in spite of this, the real responsibility for the welfare and comfort of the patients rested with the Senior House Pupil. He was in fact, if not in theory, the doctor in charge. When the Visiting Physician left the Hospital after his morning rounds, the Senior had full responsibility until the next morning.

Today when the Hospital has so many "assistant residents," plain "residents," and "chief residents" — young doctors who have completed their twelve months of service as interns and who have been selected for promotion to higher positions — it is hard to believe that in our day, there were no residents at all, that no other young men besides the house pupils were working in the hospital. The seniors in our day, on both the surgical and medical services, had a very real responsibility. George and I, however, were about the last to enjoy the old system, for under Dr. Edsall a new regime was about to be unfolded.

George was a good doctor. He knew instinctively how to take care of sick people, and he made them comfortable. His orders were explicit and complete: "This patient is to have a hot pack — wet sheet wrung out at temp. 95° so that when it reaches the patient it will be about 85°. Wrap patient in blanket for 10 minutes (repeat in 2 hrs. if awake)." For another patient he wrote: "Divide the food into six small feedings. For breakfast have the egg soft boiled and the toast well buttered. In mid-morning beef broth without too much salt, and two crackers. Do not give coarse vegetables with excessive roughage, and have the meat chopped finely and not cooked too much. Get in a glass of milk in the afternoon and again at bedtime." Imagine the house officer writing orders like that to the students of dietetics we have today!

The East and West Medical Services admitted new patients on alternate days. On the off days, each service was responsible for any medical emergencies that might be brought into the Accident Room. At any time in the twenty-four hours on the "East days" a call might come from the Accident Room: "You have a new patient just admitted," and either the Junior or the Senior would have to go down quickly. To stop whatever he was doing, even if he were attending the Ward Visit, was always an irritating interruption, but it was necessary for the running of the Hospital. Fortunately, it was often possible to give a few temporary orders and to postpone the complete study of the patient until later.

The Accident Room was actually several rooms. Across the hall from the receiving room were two smaller rooms, one with a large window to give light for minor operations, and the other the "shock room" with a "very modern" shock table, the top of which was a flat copper tank kept full of warm water so that patients in shock could be warmed up as rapidly as possible. This shock table could be tilted up or down. Unfortunately, the orderly was not always familiar with the physiology of pulmonary congestion as opposed to the physiology of cerebral anoxia and I can well remember the day when the whole Service was called to the Accident Room for an emergency. There we found our recurrent patient, S——, who suffered from severe aortic regurgitation, lying on the shock table, but head down. His face was almost black, and he was gasping for breath. George grabbed the release lever and pushed the table and the patient into the head-up position. The man gasped, took a couple of long breaths, and his color changed from blue to pink.

He began to live again. "Gosh, Dr. Minot, I thought I was gone that time. You saved my life. Thank you," he said.

Every evening up in the Flat, the Senior and Junior would "go over the books" together. More often than not the Pup would be there, too — all of us sprawled out on the Junior's bed in as comfortable positions as possible. If one of us had his "afternoon off" — that is, if conditions were such that he could leave the hospital long enough to go out to dinner — the books were gone over when he returned. Histories, physical examinations, and laboratory reports were made on loose-leaf pages, which were held in a big record book, one for each ward. To turn the pages was to review the progress of each case and to discuss the next steps in diagnosis and treatment. Could there be a better way for a young doctor to learn about medicine?

It is interesting to compare the numbers of patients and the different diseases that we had in those days with the present figures. The season of the year is always important because most of the infections, especially pneumonia, have a seasonal incidence. When one compares August and November 1913, the first and last months of George's Senior Service, with the same months in 1952, one sees first the difference in the total numbers of cases admitted to the East Medical Service.[2] The figure of 58 cases admitted in August 1913, has increased to 116 for August 1952, and for November, the figures have gone up from 79 to 127. The average age of the patients in these groups has increased from 36.0 years to 49.5 years. The average number of days spent by each patient in the Hospital has been reduced somewhat, but not as much as one might expect. In 1913, our patients stayed for an average of a little less than 14 days, whereas the present figure is down to 10.4 days.

These figures for the gross averages are misleading. In 1913, taking the months of August and November together, only 15 out of 137 (about 11 percent) of our patients stayed in the Hospital for as short a time as two days or less, while in 1952 76 out of 243 (about 31 percent) stayed for two days or less. The difference depends largely on the development of the Overnight Ward, an outgrowth of our old Accident Ward. Here the "workup" of each patient is satisfactory for practical purposes, but it is not elaborate. It includes x-ray and enough chemical tests to reach a good evaluation of the patient's problem, and so give him competent advice.

In August and in November 1913, George took care of 5 cases of typhoid fever, a disease very rare today. There were 13 cases of syphilis as against only 2 in 1952, and 7 cases of pulmonary tuberculosis as against only 1 recorded in August and November 1952. On the other hand, chronic lung disease — bronchiectasis, asthma, and emphysema — was not observed at all in 1913, at least not in those particular months, while in 1952 there were 20 cases listed. Types of cancer that were recognized 9 times in 1913 were found in 23 cases in 1952. Today both doctors and patients are more alert to the possibility of cancer and the doctors are more skillful in finding it.

The striking change is in the incidence of diseases of the heart, arteries, and kidneys. There were 8 patients in 1913 as against 60 in 1952. Evidently manual work, exercise, and walking do no harm! It is the lack of them in this modern automotive age that causes trouble, or at least the modern theory about the increase of angina pectoris and coronary thrombosis maintains this. It is curious that the disorders of digestion, of the liver, and of the blood are seen in about the same proportion today as they were before. Neurosis and neurasthenia were observed in 1913, but not nearly enough attention was paid to the reasons why they had developed, even though our teachers were practitioners of great skill and with wide experience. In 1913, the young girl who was rescued from her own mercury poisoning was transferred to the McLean Hospital, a special institution designed for the treatment of psychiatric disorders and affiliated with the Massachusetts General Hospital. There was no attempt to find out the cause of her distress before her transfer from the M.G.H., and, more important, no one worried about the very real danger of further self-injury. Today this would not happen, for there is a department of psychiatry in the M.G.H. itself, which can take care of such emergencies.

These figures listing the total cases are interesting, but they tell only part of the story. They give no idea about treatment or its results. Thanks to the advances in knowledge made by experimental researches, the nature of many diseases can now be described. This means that the treatment, which includes excellent general management, remarkable drugs, and wonderful surgery, is much more effective than before. But now, as then, it is the quality of the work that is infinitely more important than the quantity. What makes the Massachusetts General Hospital, and all the other hospitals affiliated with the Harvard Medical School, so great is the high standard that they set. The young men who work here are exposed to the theory and practice of medicine at its best.

There is another aspect of the comparison between 1913 and 1952 that is hard to overlook. In 1913, the Massachusetts General Hospital had a total of 267 beds, and the cost per patient day was only a few cents over $3.00. Forty years later, in 1953, the number of beds, exclusive of the private wards, has gone up to 528, but the cost has risen to $24.13 per patient day. In 1913, about half of the patients admitted were treated without charge. In 1952 only about 6 percent were treated free, but another 30 percent were treated part free. The extraordinary contrast between 1913 and 1952, however, is this: in 1912, the total operating cost of the Hospital was $454,531.-19, whereas in 1952 the total operating cost came to the remarkable figure of $9,733,543.67, or more than twenty times the first amount.

This remarkable increase is due to the ever-growing efficiency of medical care in hospitals everywhere: to the demand of private patients and their doctors for the centralized facilities for diagnosis and treatment. It is also the result of inflation. The Phillips House, a private building for well-to-do patients, which opened in 1917 with 94 beds, pays for itself, and the Baker Memorial Hospital, opened in 1930 with 335 beds "for people of moderate means," also pays for itself. These two units add enormously to the total operating cost of the Hospital, but they do not add to its deficit.

Advances in diagnosis and treatment have led to a tremendous expansion of all laboratories, with paid technicians doing the work that we house pupils had to do, and doing infinitely more besides. It is hard to realize that as house pupils George Minot and I knew nothing whatever about those laboratory procedures that have become so commonplace today. Such determinations as the amount of sugar in the blood, the measure of the total blood nitrogen and the nonprotein nitrogen, the measure of chlorides, sodium, and potassium are some of the tests that are made today on hundreds of patients — thanks again to our professor, Dr. Otto Folin! The results make it possible to treat our patients with much greater accuracy and efficiency. Not infrequently the abnormal figures, when discovered in time, lead to a definitive treatment that saves life. Today the new techniques of diagnosis and treatment require that three times as many people must be employed in the M.G.H. as there were in 1913. Today two-thirds of the cost is for wages and salaries; one-third is for supplies. In 1913 it was the other way around.

These figures say nothing about money spent on research. The new Research Building is supported by special grants. In the general hospital wards, careful study of complex problems is part of the routine, to be sure, but the results are available for use in clinical researches of many kinds. Without the inquisitiveness that research engenders, no one would bother to take the x-rays to look for osteoporosis, for example, and then the patient with disease unrecognized and untreated might go on to develop a "spontaneous" fracture of the spine, or perhaps of a long bone.

Research and good care of patients cannot be separated. When donors of money for research complain that some of it is being spent for patient care, they do not realize that the patient is essential, because he provides the data and the material for research. In the other direction, the result of intensive study in the laboratory is likely to help the patient and perhaps to cure him.

Back in 1912, the start of these remarkable advances was being made by Dr. Edsall. George Minot understood what was going on, and was quick to take advantage of it. He was a very competent House Pupil. He seemed to acquire knowledge and experience without effort, almost by "diffusion."

There was one patient who could have been the object of important observations (M.G.H. Case Record E.M. 190819). She had had two operations on her intestines, each resulting in the bringing of a loop of bowel up through the incision in the abdominal wall, to be easily opened and drained on the outside of the body. When George wrote on the record, "It is too bad no one here has time to carry on investigations on this case, which is an excellent opportunity," he was thinking of William Beaumont, the pioneer Army surgeon who found the half-breed Alexis St. Martin with an old gunshot wound that had resulted in a direct connection between the stomach and the outside world. Through the hole, Beaumont could follow the course of the digestive process. Beaumont was a true scientist in spite of his environment, and George Minot was sorry to have to pass up the opportunity of repeating some of his classic observations and perhaps extending them.

Because I have always been interested in asthma, I am pleased with George's notes on the following case. The patient (M.G.H. Case Record E.M. 191002) was a young woman twenty-four years of age, who had had asthma for two years, occurring in attacks at long intervals. She had been better in the mountains, and was somewhat improved in various hospitals. Orders for her treatment included the elimination of all protein from her diet, injections of adrenalin 1–1000, 15 minims at a dose. George notes: "The blood pressure is low — it is curious that with the increased intrapulmonary pressure the blood pressure is not higher." And then follows a note that was written by George Minot on September 26, 1913, a year after Schloss's description of the egg-sensitive child, but before Walker's studies on asthma and before Cook's description of horse asthma: "Two days ago, inoculation like a Von Pirquet with egg albumin — no reaction. We intended to carry out a series of such inoculations with crude protein substances for ideas of what may cause anaphylaxis [sensitivity reaction] in reference to her asthma."

George was in close touch with the progress of medicine as it is described from week to week and month to month in the medical journals. His desire to correlate anaphylaxis and asthma was not only abreast of the literature; it was ahead of it. If this study could have been made, he might have discovered the cause of the trouble in that case, and so developed an understanding of the allergic diseases.

Aside from the routine laboratory tests, there was remarkably little in the way of investigation as we know it today. Nephritis was treated with a salt-free diet, as well as with injections of theocin, helped out by hot packs. Exophthalmic goiter was treated symptomatically with rest, and good food, and with what today is known as "T.L.C." (tender loving care). The determination of the rate of basal metabolism as an index of the function of the thyroid gland was soon to be made possible and practical by the researches of Dr. Eugene F. Dubois in New York, and of Dr. James H. Means[3] in

Boston (Dr. Means had been Senior when George was Pup), but the test for B.M.R. was not available in 1913. We had no sulfa drugs, and, of course, no antibiotics. It was thirty years before penicillin was made available, in 1942. We had no intravenous fluids, no blood transfusions, and we did not know about the use of oxygen in treatment.

X-rays were beginning to be appreciated. The morning visit was apt to include a trip to the X-ray Department, and there was Dr. Walter J. Dodd, a thin spare man, with his face pocked by x-ray burns and scarred from the plastic operations on it. His hands were badly burned, the fingers partly gone. He wore gloves to hide the deformity. What a charming, delightful man he was! His enthusiasm was contagious, and to hear him explain and discuss his plates,* with anecdotes and funny but pertinent stories interjected, was as entertaining as it was instructive. With him was his assistant, Dr. George W. Holmes, a "Down-Easter," who later inherited Dr. Dodd's position, as well as most of his qualities and abilities, and who became friend and teacher to us all.

The X-ray Department occupied two small rooms just beyond the Accident Room. The larger room had a brick fireplace, which made it an attractive place to gather. We could smoke as we listened to the experts. The Surgical Visitors were often there at the same time, looking at broken bones while we looked at stomachs and chests. Barium enemas were not used until later, which is interesting, since the procedure is harmless. Our patients with peptic ulcer were referred promptly to the Surgical Service. There was no attempt to treat them medically, and the difference in symptoms, in treatment, and in prognosis between lesions in front of the pylorus, the outlet of the stomach, and lesions beyond it were not clarified. Ulcers of the stomach require operation much more often than ulcers of the duodenum, the part of the intestine beyond the pylorus. Most of our patients were operated on, but, curiously, the end results were never discussed by the Medical Service. Was this because we House Pupils, as well as our Visiting Physician, were too busy to walk over to the surgical ward to see what had happened to our old patient-friend, or did we have such faith in the surgeons as

* These early x-rays were taken on glass plates. Even in World War I, overseas, the x-rays that looked for bullets and shrapnel were taken on glass plates.

to know that the patient would be all right under their care? Our system of clinical records was partly responsible for this apparent neglect. When the patient was transferred to the Surgical Service, a brand new record had to be made, beginning with the history, just as if the patient had been moved to another hospital. In our day, the line drawn between medicine and surgery was much too sharp, and there was not nearly enough discussion and coöperation between the two Services. Today all that has been corrected, to the great advantage of all concerned.

In the Out-Patient Department this compartmentalization was complete. Notes were made on cards that were different for each clinic, and no attention was paid to the sequence of visits or to the over-all progress of the patient. When the patient was sent into the ward, these O.P.D. cards had to be summarized by the Junior or the Pup, and then for the first time some order and sense was made out of them. The record of hospitalization ended when the patient left the Service, and it was bound separately. The consulting surgeon had no chance to look over this record, for his House Pupil summarized only the salient points, and then later the surgical record also was filed separately. When the patient left the hospital and came back once more to the Out-Patient Department, the entire House record, both medical and surgical, was ignored, unless perhaps the House Officer was enterprising and energetic enough to look up the various parts of it in the Record Room, and usually that was just too much trouble. The establishment of Unit Records on January 1, 1937 was indeed a step forward. Since then, everything that happens to the patient in any department of the Hospital at any time is recorded chronologically on pages bound together between the covers of a single folder, and the understanding of the patient as a whole has improved tremendously.

On November 30, 1913, George's service as House Pupil at the Massachusetts General Hospital was completed. On that day I was to become Senior. When I returned from a two weeks' vacation, all ready to take his place, the Transfer Visit was made, and George turned over to my care all his patients in a ceremony which to us was impressive. At about 5 P.M., the five of us on the service met in the Flat, and then we made a complete visit to all the East Medical patients. At each bed we stopped, and George explained to me, the new Senior, the chief points about each — a quick review of the history, the interesting findings on examination, and then a brief survey of the treatment. George's parting from each ward was quite sad. All the nurses were devoted to the patients, and under Dr. George Minot they had learned much about patient care. They had seen his devotion to all those under his charge, and his exemplary behavior and attitudes had impressed them. They were sorry to lose his leadership. George, in turn, knew how hard the nurses had worked. Each morning and evening he had gone around with them to hear their reports and to discuss the next steps. He was grateful indeed for their interest and their support, not to mention the many things that he had learned from them.

The trip through the lower wards was easier; there were only one or two East Medical patients in each one, and the nurse was interested in other services besides ours. Just the same, George was grateful to them, and sorry to leave, and the nurses and patients were sorry to have him go.

Back in the Flat, someone found a bottle, and each of us had just enough to drink the others' healths. George took off his white suit and changed to his "city clothes," just like a bride going away. At the bottom of the Flat stairs, a wheelchair was waiting; George got in, someone carried his bag, we pushed him through the Brick Corridor and out through the Bulfinch Building. Meanwhile, the West Medical Service had been holding its own Transfer Visit, and Orville Rogers, their retiring Senior, was in another wheelchair. The two of them left together in Tom Lee's hack. We watched them disappear around the corner.

5

Baltimore

What should we do after our service as House Pupil at the Massachusetts General Hospital? None of us took the time — indeed, we did not have the time — to think very much about the question until toward the end. There were two principal possibilities; the obvious one was to open an office and begin the practice of medicine without further procrastination; the other was to learn more about the science of medicine by investigating a problem in research.

When George Minot graduated from the Medical School, the study of medicine was changing. Even before Dr. Edsall came to the Massachusetts General Hospital in the spring of 1912, the young men, and their clinical teachers, too, had begun to realize that if the many observations about individual patients could be put together, some new principles might be found. In those days, research was being conducted only in the basic sciences — in anatomy, pathology, and physiology.

What about research in the hospital — at the bedside? Was it not possible to study such simple matters as the blood pressure or the blood cells? Why were not those simple studies "research" just as much as were the more complex problems of nutrition or chemistry? Were not Dr. Roger I. Lee, Assistant Physician, and young Dr. Paul D. White, House Pupil on the West Medical Service at the Massachusetts General Hospital, making a useful contribution when they described a simple technique[1] for determining the speed of blood coagulation? Dr. Walter W. Palmer and Dr. James L. Gamble, recent House Pupils, were making progress under the stimulation of Professor Lawrence J. Henderson in studying the balance of acids and bases in the body. The general idea was beginning to take hold, but it came slowly.

Dr. Reginald Fitz, writing his reminiscences for Dr. Washburn's History of the Massachusetts General Hospital, said: "I remember when I was a House Officer [in 1910–11] that the Interurban Club [a group of important physicians from various cities] was to meet . . . and there was nothing new going on in the M.G.H. that could be of any possible interest to the type of man who belonged to the Interurban Club . . . The program . . . was devoted entirely to [a discussion of] teaching methods." [2]

When Dr. Edsall came, the idea of research was discussed more than ever. George Minot was much interested in patients with diseases of the blood, but his routine work was so overwhelming that little could be accomplished beyond improving his clinical impressions. He did find time to publish with Dr. L. Harry Newburgh a paper[3] that showed that the blood pressure in pneumonia became lower as the patient became sicker. He was also keeping notes on special cases, to be useful later.

Libraries and books are essential tools in research. The investigator must keep his eye on the current literature to see what others are observing in similar cases. To read the papers published in medical journals is essential; but to go to medical meetings and to hear the investigator present his findings is better, especially if one can meet the speaker after the formal session to discuss the matter and to compare notes face to face.

When George talked with Dr. Edsall about his future, Dr. Edsall recommended that he go away from Boston if possible, and find work in a new place under the best possible instructor. George would find a different way of doing things, and perhaps a different atmosphere, which might rearrange his thoughts and perhaps add a new idea.

The Medical School of Johns Hopkins University was young. Dr. William Osler's influence was still felt there, even though the Master had left Baltimore to become the Regius Professor of Medicine at Oxford. Dr. William H. Welch, another of the four great founders of the Johns Hopkins Medical School, was still active in his pathology laboratory, stimulating young men to think about the possible mechanisms of disease. At Johns Hopkins, progress was being made in learning new methods which would improve both the diagnosis of disease and the treatment of patients. The atmosphere in Baltimore was scientific, and it was stimulating.

If George could go to Johns Hopkins for a year or two, the time would be well spent, Dr. Edsall said, and he added that he would be pleased to write to Dr. Thayer to see whether there might be a place for George Minot at Johns Hopkins.

Dr. William Sidney Thayer was Clinical Professor of Medicine at Johns Hopkins. He was a clinician of great ability, an excellent teacher, and a charming person. He was the important consultant in medicine in Baltimore. He dressed immaculately — I can remember the black-and-white checked suit, which fitted so well, and the heavy-rimmed pince-nez eyeglasses on the end of a long black silk ribbon with which he used to twirl his glasses whenever he was thinking about something.

Dr. Thayer was well known in Boston. Some of his family lived there. He was a great friend of Dr. Frederick C. Shattuck, his counterpart in Boston, and was much like him, even to the flower in his buttonhole.

One person who encouraged George to go to Hopkins was Dr. Francis W. Peabody. He was four years older than George, and since the Minots and the Peabodys knew each other as families, so George had met Francis on numerous occasions. Francis had been an M.G.H. House Pupil, and after that, he had been one of the first to be invited to Baltimore to gain additional experience under Dr. Thayer. Dr. Reginald Fitz followed Peabody in 1911. After Fitz, Dr. Thayer had chosen Dr. Roy R. Snowden, a Hopkins graduate. These were outstanding young men, and it was not surprising that Dr. Thayer should invite the next outstanding young man — Dr. George Minot — to follow them.

Dr. Edsall's letter had told Dr. Thayer about George, but it was not really necessary, for Dr. Thayer knew about him anyway; he knew his father, and he knew George's Cousin Charles, the Medical School professor. Dr. Thayer was delighted at the prospect of having George come to work with him in Baltimore.

Even though George appreciated the compliment of the invitation quite thoroughly, he was not sure that he wanted to go. He had never been away from his family and alone in a strange place for any length of time. He was tired after his hospital service, and he feared that his general health might not be good enough to stand a different way of life in a new environment. His father, as well as Francis Peabody, encouraged him, and, just as in his decision about the Medical School, he knew instinctively that he would go. On Monday, December 22, 1913, he and I dined together at the Harvard Club in Boston, and we "opened wine," seeking consolation and maybe a little sympathy, if not wisdom, from the bottle. The decision was made quickly; the letter to Dr. Thayer was dispatched, and on Friday, December 26, I lunched at 188 and said goodbye. Cousin Jim saw George off that evening.

The New Year, 1914, saw George in Baltimore. As expected, he was lonely, but fortunately he was busy. On January 3, he wrote me at some length. He said among other things:

> Snowed under with work — Two internes: one sick and "little me" has been given the job to run the duties of Senior, Junior, Pup, and Sub-Pup on 18 patients and had 2 admissions today. Also have 6 private cases of Dr. T's to care for . . . Charts, drugs, every last thing is utterly different . . . I act as a regular resident over the 2 house officers and the colored ward which holds about 24 patients.

That the first impression George made on his contemporaries was good may be gathered from an excellent "Recollection" sent me by Dr. Roy Snowden:

> For several months Dr. Thayer had frequently referred to the approaching advent of "Minot" (we rather scorned the use of first names in those manly days), and the glowing reference by the chief and the fact that "Minot" was an illustrious name in medicine, built up in our minds the idea that we were about to meet a paragon of overwhelming dignity. This conception dissolved instantly when I first met George, for his greeting was a rare combination of friendliness and modesty, almost to the point of humility. We never had occasion to reverse that first impression, for George was so fundamentally kind and thoughtful that we all instinctively took him into our innermost circle of close friendship.[4]

George's letter to me continues:

> I have a room bigger than at 188. The bath is 25 yards away . . . There is no "Mollie," only a rather poor, inefficient, colored maid, so

that when the wash comes up you have to put it away yourself! . . . Food is not unlike M.G.H. . . . There is no ice box or crackers in the living room and no fireplace — only daily papers and a "graphaphone" . . . People seldom there.

My duties are 1) Care of private cases — 7 at present . . . 2) Supervise the interne on colored ward — perhaps suggest this or that and he reports things to me. This is fun and no work. 3) Monday 9–11 hold Dr. T's hand on rounds, same on Wed. Wed. 10–1 Clinic and one on Thurs. Thursday 10–12 work with Dr. T. in the O.P.D. — Later on I believe I am to help teach a student or two. 4) Later shall do some special work.

Dr. Snowden has amplified the story:

George's duties as Dr. Thayer's assistant were many and varied. In addition to having professional charge of the chief's private room patients, he was responsible for the itinerary of the teaching ward rounds, and also for the selection of the patients in Dr. Thayer's weekly clinic. These routine duties took up most of each morning and a good part of three or four afternoons. The assistant had another important responsibility, which was to hover constantly at the side of [Dr. Thayer] . . . ready to tactfully get him down out of the clouds of an enthusiastic and prolonged dissertation on some rare clinical sign, and also to pick up the stethoscope, the ophthalmoscope, and nose glasses (including the silk cord), the wrist watch, the handkerchief (which was carried tucked under the wrist watch), and any other of the numerous and sundry personal objects that could be detached and laid on the bed and then completely forgotten. George and I often met before dinner for a brief review of the chief's idiosyncrasies of that day, and the opportunity thus given for full play of George's kindly wit was more diverting and relaxing than a cocktail.

Dr. Alan M. Chesney, who was the assistant resident physician assigned to look after the private patients of Dr. Lewellys F. Barker, the Professor of Medicine, writes me:

We had our living quarters in the main administration building, the one with the big dome that forms such a landmark in Baltimore . . . [George and I] used to take one another's calls on the not very frequent occasions when one or the other of us could manage to get an evening off from our work.

George was well liked by all of the men on the resident staff who knew him. Indeed, he got to know many of his fellow residents very well for he never held himself aloof from the rest of us but, on the contrary, appeared eager to seek acquaintanceship with this new group of young Hopkins physicians with whom he had been thrown, and did not hesitate to join the group when it repaired to the nearby tavern of Louis Hanselmann for a glass of beer when the evening's work was done.

He was also interested in seeing something of life in Maryland and asked me on one occasion if I would introduce him to some of my friends. Of course I was glad to do so and can recall vividly two Sundays that he and I spent together in two homes in Baltimore County in the spring of 1914.

When George arrived in Baltimore . . . it was Dr. Thayer's intention to put him to work on a problem connected with the circulation, as I recall it, but George's interest in the blood had already developed and since the late Dr. William H. Howell, who was then Professor of Physiology in the School of Medicine, was at work on the problem of the coagulation of the blood, it was natural that George should seek the opportunity to work with Dr. Howell . . . I recall that years later at a dinner in Baltimore in his honor, George referred to this circumstance and expressed some misgiving lest he might have offended Dr. Thayer in not following out his wishes by working on the problem which had been suggested to him . . . Dr. Thayer, who was present, lost no time in saying that, far from being offended, he had been instead delighted to have an assistant who already knew what problem he wanted to work on.

George's physical appearance in that year of his stay at Hopkins was already indicative of what it would be in later years. Tall, thin, slightly stoop-shouldered, his hair already thinning . . . he would never appear to be really robust, and that is how matters turned out. But he did his work as assistant resident physician faithfully and well and when he left the Hopkins environment to return to his native New England he left many friends behind who respected and admired him and were genuinely fond of him. Indeed, the Hopkins medical institutions have always regarded him as a foster son and always took the greatest pride in the distinction which he later achieved.

On Friday, January 9, George's letter to me was cheerful:

Last night dance here at hospital. Met a raft of people . . . and I got in with the right crowd I guess, as beer, food, and whiskey appeared in one of the fellow's rooms and he asked me to join and you bet I did — bed at 2 A.M. Mrs. Thayer took me round and introduced me to her group. A bit sleepy today, but I see I can take a nap now from 3–5:30, then see patients, dress and go to [debutante] assembly with dinner at the DeL's at 8 P.M. and probably back about 3 A.M. Sounds just like M.G.H. hospital life? — Does it? — It does not . . . Dr. Smith and Dr. Norton front door officials are delightful and very cordial. They introduced themselves to me. Were great leaders at the ball last night.

George wanted me to join him in Baltimore:

Jan. 20: I spoke to Dr. Thayer about you. He says that if you care to come here to see how it is done in other places than Boston, you could step in under Whipple pathologist age 35 ± who is carrying on very interesting experimental pathological lesions in animals on liver disease and functions. Whipple said he could work you in well.

This was the Dr. George H. Whipple who was destined to share the Nobel Prize with Dr. George R. Minot in 1934. At that time he was working with Dr. Welch.

It was typical of George to worry about me; to try to help me:

Feb. 1. I wonder if Dr. Edsall has talked with you yet. I think I know what he is to talk about . . . Write me what he says. I heard here about the M.G.H. H.O. exams from Dr. Thayer the day before your letters. How he gets such news — Lord knows! Last night dined at the C's and after dinner to a dance at Mrs. F's — all very swell . . . Before that I hadn't been out since Sunday when I went calling on those who have been polite . . . Feel as if I was learning lots and yet again what an easy day as compared with M.G.H.

Feb. 13. I find I am getting very narrow — my general knowledge of other things than wards and patients seems perfectly nil, especially as compared with the men here. You see they all have a lot of lab diagnosis and training. I have found next to nothing that I know that they don't and they know a million things I never dreamed of. It is not so much what you do here as it is what you see, hear, and meet, etc.

And then he described a series of social events — dinners, theater parties, suppers, dances — he was lonely no longer!

In late February, I had been talking with Dr. Edsall about my own plans, and he had urged me to go to work with Dr. Warfield T. Longcope, Bard Professor of Medicine at Columbia and Chief of Medicine at the Presbyterian Hospital in New York — if Dr. Longcope would take me. Dr. Longcope was interested in immunology and anaphylaxis. George was enthusiastic about my plans.

One Saturday night I broke away from my M.G.H. patients and went to New York on the midnight train to see Dr. Longcope on Sunday morning. He offered me a job, and I accepted it, to begin the first of May. George wrote me:

[The results of your visit with Dr.] Longcope interest me greatly . . . How much will you see Longcope? Will there be several other men working in the same lab? I understand Longcope is excellent, it sounds good to me. I should think knowledge about asthma, etc., would be good. It would in the end mean that you tried to find the cause and then the prevention or cure. But of course the problems take you well afield before reaching the real end — like everything else as far as I can see. I do feel that work with Longcope of any sort — to see new men, new hospitals, get in with American medicine, etc., is advantageous. When you come here, I will tell you about a speech which Dr. Thayer delivered to a bunch of residents here one night at dinner . . . I hate the idea of New York as New York, but this is foolish, because after you have been there for a month all will be fine. I strongly believe it is an excellent opportunity.

These letters reveal an important, vital side of George's character. Although some of us are not much interested in the plans of others — thinking, perhaps, that it is their business and not ours, and that we should express our opinion only when invited to do so — George Minot had the other idea. His interest was active. Success in his work and recognition by his superiors had given him an increasing self-confidence. There was no thought of intruding, but always he was looking to see how his associates could improve their status, or perhaps their work, by taking the right step. In my case especially he was concerned quite sincerely with my welfare, and he tried hard to steer me to the right track. Later on he was to steer many others in the same way.

Another thing about his letters is their reference to people: "It is not so much what you do as what you see, hear, and meet." Having begun to understand himself, he was learning to recognize the difference between a good man and a poor one, and he tried to associate with the best. Dr. Edsall's advice about a change of scene had been wise.

In February, George's own future was beginning to disturb him: "Official job here ends October 1, but I'll probably be here till Dec. 1 — or so." And then incidentally, he wondered how he was going to get away for the meeting of the "Edgartown High School" at Chappaquiddick on April 17.

My service as Senior House Pupil at the Massachusetts General Hospital ended on March 31. In the next three days, I did nothing but sleep and eat. On Friday, April 3, Dr. George P. Denny and I took the Federal Express to Baltimore to visit George.

On Saturday morning he showed Denny and me all over the

Johns Hopkins Hospital, through "miles" of corridors and up and down stairs. The open wards at the ends of short passageways were different from our wards at home, and the two or three single rooms opening off the passageway were useful for the easy isolation of any patient who needed special attention. Today the arrangement of the wards in new hospitals is quite like the old scheme at "the Hopkins."

Dr. Barker's Saturday clinic at noon was impressive; everybody attended and heard this excellent clinician discuss his cases. Denny and I met many of George's associates. On Monday and Tuesday we made rounds with Dr. Thayer and then lunched with him at the Maryland Club — "very swell," as my diary says.

We three had dinner with Dr. L. G. Rowntree, who was working on the kidney. He was looking for young men to work with him. The opportunity was good, but we were pretty well committed to other arangements. George Minot had no desire to change the direction of his interest.

On May 1, I began my own work with Dr. Longcope in New York. Six weeks later, George returned from Baltimore. My sister was to marry Edward Wigglesworth, George's classmate who had gone to Europe with him. We who were to be ushers dined together on Saturday night, June 13, 1914. It was what George called a "large evening." In the week of the wedding came the Harvard Commencement, with its many social activities, and we took in some of them. On Monday, June 22, George and I went by day train to the meeting of the American Medical Association in Atlantic City. George knew it would be "good for us." We attended the President's Ball and listened to papers by men some of whose names were beginning to be a little familiar.

In July, George had to return to Baltimore, while I spent the month at "Chappy." Later in the month George caught an infection and was miserable. He was expected to work during August also, because several other men were out on account of illness, but Dr. Thayer recognized his poor condition, and, after a few days' observation in the private ward, he changed all the plans so that George could be off entirely for the rest of the summer. On August 4, on his way home, George stopped in New York, and we had dinner and spent the evening together. Incidentally, it took three letters and a postcard to make sure that I understood the time and place of our meeting. George looked tired and washed out; the infection had evidently been severe. But the coast of Maine is a place where exhausted people are restored to health easily and successfully, and after a week at North Haven, George wrote: "Am better than ever, sunburnt, gained weight and seem fine. Delightful crowd here . . . Tennis each A.M. and sail each P.M. . . . Barbara H. created excitement by going to pool in skin-tight short-sleeved and leg bathing suit."

The *Dorel* had been sold, but George was invited to go cruising on other boats, and all was well. One letter describes a pleasant day on a schooner, with a number of boys and girls — one girl being Marian Linzee Weld, who had belonged to George's "army" in the early days at Bar Harbor. The last letter of the season says: "Sept. 12, 1914: On board the 'Lady Mary' off Bass Harbor Bar. I don't believe I will ever work again, and have quite forgotten how to speak medicine."

In late September, George went back to Baltimore, and this time his life was quite different. He was now in Dr. Howell's laboratory, working full time on his problems with the blood.

Earlier in the year, there had been a patient with pernicious anemia on Dr. Thayer's ward, and George had shown unusual interest in his problem. Careful and complete studies had been made, especially of the nitrogen metabolism. The decision to remove the man's spleen provided the opportunity to study the metabolism before and after operation. It was found that splenectomy stopped the loss of nitrogen from the body, and that improvement in the patient's general condition, as well as in his blood picture, coincided with the restoration of a positive nitrogen balance.[5]

When, later on, Dr. Thayer talked with Dr. Howell about his young assistant, who was so well grounded in his knowledge of blood and so eager to apply what he knew, Dr. Howell was quite ready to give George a place in his laboratory.

Dr. Howell was "a wise old man and an excellent teacher," as George Denny describes him, and he had written one of the best textbooks in English on physiology. He was a typical professor — quiet, dignified, devoted to his work and confined to his laboratory

— but he also knew about human nature as he found it in young men.

Dr. Howell introduced Minot and Denny to organized physiological research. His theory of blood coagulation was that the fibrin which makes blood clot is formed when its precursor, fibrinogen, is acted upon by an enzyme called thrombin. This thrombin in turn comes from a mother substance, prothrombin. There were two theories to explain why blood outside of the blood vessels does clot and why blood inside of the vessels does not clot. The older theory of Morowitz held that when the tissues were injured and blood escaped, the tissues released an enzyme, "thrombokinase," which in the presence of calcium converted the prothrombin into thrombin and so produced the clot. Dr. Howell was working on a slightly different theory. He could show that, in addition to prothrombin, blood contained an antithrombin to inhibit the prothrombin until another substance derived from the blood platelets — he called it "thromboplastin" — removed the antithrombin. When blood was shed this thromboplastin was released from the blood itself. Dr. Howell showed that prothrombin could be isolated and stored as a dry powder, readily soluble in a weak solution of sodium bicarbonate. When prothrombin solution was added to fibrinogen in the presence of calcium, a clot formed — the calcium converted the prothrombin into thrombin — but this happened only in case antithrombin was not present.

Antithrombin could not be isolated as such at that time, but its presence could be estimated by the fact that venous blood, taken as it came away from different organs of the body, varied considerably in its ability to inhibit the clot in prothrombin-calcium-fibrinogen mixtures.

The upshot of the work was the finding that antithrombin came from the liver, and that more of it came if the circulation to the liver was impeded so as to produce congestion.[6] Other organs produced very little antithrombin, even if their circulation was slowed. These findings explain why it is that the coagulation of the blood is altered in certain diseases of the liver. The studies begun by Minot and Denny under Dr. Howell's guidance led to studies by other men in the same laboratory, and from them to Dr. Howell's discovery and isolation of the anticoagulant "heparin," which has the properties of the original antithrombin. Heparin is used today in many laboratory experiments, and sometimes in the treatment of patients when the clotting of blood must be prevented, as in operations on the heart or on arteries.

Dr. Roy R. Snowden adds an amusing incident, which shows that George's hands were not nearly so good as his head. He writes:

> George's technical activities in the laboratory were carried out with his characteristic restless energy, and not infrequently his haste in setting up some intricate apparatus would result in a crash of glassware, whereupon there would be heard a high-pitched series of witty expletives that would convulse us all and release George of any pent-up frustration. This aspect of his laboratory career at Hopkins reached its climax early one Sunday morning when George was working all alone in the deserted laboratory building. A ten-gallon demijohn of pure alcohol caught fire and rapidly turned into a fiery fountain. When the raging conflagration had been subdued by the city fire department, George's innate sense of humor was still functioning as he described to me how he rushed to the laboratory door and cheerily called out into the empty hall, "A little help, please."

For George, the hard part was not the handling of the laboratory animals or the chemical manipulations by which the various fractions were separated from the different blood samples; the hard part was the writing of the papers. He was particular about every detail; every measurement had to be checked again and again, and every word in the description had to be just right. His command of English was not quite up to his other abilities; he had difficulty in writing down exactly what he wanted to say. When his sentences were clumsy, or perhaps ambiguous, he was slow to accept suggestions for improvement. The result was that the preparation of papers was much more difficult than it should have been. Later, his wife was to help him greatly with his writing. To her comments and criticisms he would listen, and then he would change the words and phrases without much argument.

In Baltimore, George became aware of another discovery — this one of a totally different kind. After the start of his second year there, I did not hear from him for some time, but on November 13 I went to Baltimore, where he met me at the station. He had a new look in his eye, something I had not seen before. He acted queerly, too; he was in a very gay mood. He was not at all disturbed about how we were going to find a cab to take us and my bag to the hotel. Nothing was said about my transportation back to New York. He showed not the slightest interest in or anxiety about these details, which usually were of considerable importance to him.

"Rack," he said, "come over here and smoke a cigarette. I have something to tell you."

I had seen that same look and that same change of personality in other friends in the past year or two, and the reason for it flashed before me all at once. "Girls?" I thought to myself. "Why, George has never even looked at the same girl twice so far as I know." I began to think of one or two vague possibilities, but I couldn't believe that there was anything doing with any of them, and finally I thought to myself, "Maybe it isn't that, anyway!" I tried not to show what I was thinking about.

"Something important?" I asked.

"Yes," said he. "Do you remember my letter about the schooner? One young lady who was on board has come down to Baltimore several times this fall to stay with the Dennys." And then he took a long breath and blurted out: "It was Marian Linzee Weld, and I am engaged to her!"

That was certainly wonderful news. Surprised? Of course I was surprised. I had no idea that any such courtship was going on, and I found later that Denny did not know of it, either. We agreed that Minot was a pretty sly old fox and pretty clever about keeping his secret.

George Denny and I knew all about Marian; we had known her all our lives. She was the daughter of Mr. Christopher Minot Weld, a man of importance in the textile business of New England. Mr. Weld's father, Francis Minot Weld, was the man who had been so closely associated with George's grandfather, George Richards Minot. George himself had known Marian since childhood; she was one of the little girls in the cottage next door at Bar Harbor, and her family lived in Boston and Milton. She was a distant cousin, besides.

Denny and I knew immediately that both George and Marian had chosen well. They had many interests in common. They loved nature — especially the deep woods at Bar Harbor — and Marian could talk well about the beautiful things that they met as they walked along. She was less shy than George, she was friendly and gracious with people, and she was destined to give George the support and sense of security that he needed. To say that we were pleased was putting it mildly. The dinner at the Dennys' house that night was a gay one. We drank to the health of Marian and George with the greatest pleasure.

Next morning we went to "the Hopkins" as usual, meeting still more men. On Monday, George and I made rounds with Dr. Thayer and attended the clinicopathological conference presided over by Dr. Welch; I left for New York at 6:35 P.M.

On Sunday, December 20, George started for Boston, traveling with the Dennys, but I lunched with him in New York between trains. His engagement was to be announced at an afternoon tea and reception at the Welds' house on the Sunday after Christmas, and the details about that required discussion.

The engagement tea and reception was a pleasant gathering of a few close friends. Marian looked lovely in a new blue dress, with the corsage from George held with a ribbon to her shoulder. She was smiling and gracious to everybody, and her mother and her two sisters were smiling and gracious, too. George was handsome, with his suit freshly pressed, his new red tie, and a large white carnation in his lapel. He was somewhat ill at ease, having to stand there to endure the critical eyes of the distinguished company. His friends did what they could to ease the strain, for the poor fellow was in a spot that was somewhat difficult for him. However, he bore up well, and he and Marian were quite aware that the congratulations were heartfelt and sincere. George's days in Baltimore were done.

In January 1915, George was back in Boston. I was still in New York. On January 28, he came to New York to see various men about their studies in blood disease. Private practice was discussed, but a new project interested him more.

Dr. Edsall had a patient with trichinosis, who had a cough due to severe bronchitis, and Dr. Edsall wanted to support his theory that the bronchitis was part of the trichinosis. His theory ran as follows: The trichina worm lives in the muscles of hogs. When infected pork is eaten by man, the larvae penetrate into the mucous membrane of the intestine and go into the blood vessels, and through them to all parts of the body. If the larvae should lodge in the bronchial tree, they could irritate it in a mechanical manner. Does this really happen, and if it does, how often?

The question looked like a good one, and quite easy to solve, especially as George and I now had access to the records of three different hospitals. If I looked up all the cases of trichinosis in the Presbyterian Hospital in New York, George could look up the cases at Johns Hopkins and the Massachusetts General Hospital, and then we could pool our results. In due course, a total of 102 records of patients with trichinosis were reviewed, and the fact that 8.8 percent of them had respiratory symptoms, severe enough to lead to the consideration of a purely pulmonary condition as the main diagnosis, was good enough to justify the effort. Needless to say, the collection of data and its arrangement into the form of a paper led to a large correspondence, concerned mostly with the details of English composition and its arrangement. Finally, however, the paper was published under the title "Respiratory Signs and Symptoms in Trichinosis." [7]

World War I had been going on for a year, but as yet it had not made any changes in our lives. Suddenly on Friday, May 7, 1915, the *Lusitania* was sunk by a German submarine, and that was a shock to everybody. America began to wake up, and President Wilson talked about military training, even though until then he had been "too proud to fight."

In June 1915, George came out to Readville, and he and I discussed the war with my father, to see what the future might have in store for us. Other Americans had begun to take active parts. Dr. Harvey Cushing had organized a Harvard Surgical Unit to serve at the American Hospital at Neuilly in Paris, and a number of our friends went with him. Dr. Robert B. Osgood had invited our classmate, Philip D. Wilson, to help him set up an orthopedic unit in England. It was not easy to sit by doing business as usual at home, and the sinking of the *Lusitania* made us more restless than ever. My father advised us to "keep our shirts on," at least for the time being. Cousin Jim, of course, felt much the same way, only more so, because he knew that George was too dependent on proper food and care to stand the rigors of any military regime. George's brothers Jimmy and Henry spent the summers of 1915, 1916, and 1917 at the military training camp that Major General Leonard Wood had organized at Plattsburg, New York, and which became in 1917 a regular Officers' Training Camp and part of the U. S. Army.

George's wedding day was not far off. Through all of June, he was busy. Life was exciting. Too many things were going on all at once. The wedding presents were coming in, and George went over to the Welds' house every night to see them — silver, china, glass, books, clocks, pictures, everything! "Why, Rack, it looks like a branch of Bigelow Kennard's store." George didn't quite know what to make of it all, but Marian was very methodical; she had a list of everything and was busy writing "thank-you" notes.

Meantime, there were many details: what color ties should the ushers wear? Should we have light-gray gloves, or dark-gray? George got their tickets for the train to Maine, but he hadn't any idea how he was going to get from Milton to the North Station at that time of day. The minister had to be met at the station in Milton, and then we had to send him back to town later. The Reverend Palfrey Perkins, Harvard '05, was a great friend of George's and Marian's, and everyone was pleased when he agreed to perform the marriage ceremony.

George gave his Ushers' Dinner at the Hoosic Whisick Club on Saturday night, June 26, and it was quite a party. When the champagne came on, everyone was happy. The first toast was, of course, "To the Bride," and after "bottoms up" the glasses were smashed in the big fireplace so that no other toast could contaminate them. Next morning we all felt a bit "brittle."

On Tuesday, June 29, 1915, George Richards Minot was married to Marian Linzee Weld in the Unitarian Church in Milton. Marian looked lovely in her white dress of satin and tulle, with orange blossoms in her hair. She was accompanied by her two sisters, Elizabeth and Margaret, as bridesmaids. I was the best man, and the ushers were George's two brothers Jimmy and Henry, Marian's two brothers, Francis Minot Weld and John Linzee Weld, Denny, Homans, Perry, and Harding, members of the "Edgartown High School," Bob Amory, and George's cousin Henry Lawrence Whitney. It was a lovely summer day, and the reception in the large house of Mr. and Mrs. Weld on Milton Street was attended by a host of friends. It was very much a gala occasion, and when at last George and Marian were driven away, everyone agreed that they were an ideal couple who would go far and accomplish much.

6

Research at M.G.H. and Huntington

When George Minot came back from Baltimore in January 1915, Dr. Edsall had been Professor of Medicine in the Harvard Medical School and Chief of Medical Services at the Massachusetts General Hospital for three years. Changes in the treatment of patients and in the teaching of students were plain for all to see. The atmosphere had a critical, scientific fragrance not present before.

Dr. James H. Means, who had been East Medical House Pupil two steps ahead of George, had been away, too. He had been studying in Europe and in New York and on return had set up the apparatus to measure respiration in the small triangular room under the out-patient amphitheater. He was beginning to measure the rate of metabolism — the speed at which our body machines run. Dr. Paul D. White had been in London, working with Sir Thomas Lewis, and had brought back a Cambridge electrocardiograph, a new instrument to study the heartbeat, and had installed it in the basement under the Skin Ward G in what he recalls now as "a little closet next to the syphilitic bathroom." Dr. Edsall had advised others besides George Minot to seek other instructors, to broaden their outlook, and to bring home new methods and new ideas.

When Dr. Otto Folin, our chemistry professor, wanted to study his new methods "at the bedside," Dr. Edsall had been pleased to help him find a place for a laboratory in a sort of loft — a large empty space over the powerhouse — and to make suitable alterations in it. Dr. Folin assigned his assistant, Dr. Willey Denis, a woman as substantial in her knowledge as in her person, to organize and run the new laboratory. A little later Dr. Lawrence J. Henderson wanted Dr. Walter W. Palmer and Dr. James L. Gamble to study the equilibria of acids and bases and the intricacies of hydrogen ions, and a nice big chemical laboratory was just what they required. They appropriated some of Dr. Denis's new domain.

These were important developments. In 1914 for the first time doctors other than House Pupils and Visiting Physicians were working in the Hospital, and in view of what goes on today that simple fact is noteworthy. These men had a purpose that was even more significant than the care of the sick patient: they were trying to learn about disease in order to discover better methods of treatment. One need hardly say that their mere presence in the Hospital made everyone more alert to observe the variations in their patients. New methods were coming, by which at least some of these variations could be actually measured and recorded in figures. The science of medicine was developing fast.

What started these new developments? Was it all due to the genius of Dr. David L. Edsall? It was tempting to think so, in the beginning, and there is no doubt that it was Dr. Edsall who did more than any other man to promote clinical research at the Massachusetts General Hospital. It was he who wanted to extend and improve the training and experience of his young men. It was he who helped to start their investigation and who encouraged them, and finally it was he who "sold" the idea to the Director and to the Trustees of the Hospital, so that his young scientists could find little places here and there to set up their laboratories and have a little money for apparatus and supplies.

It was natural for us to think that the Massachusetts General Hospital was far ahead of her sister institutions in this development, but it was soon realized that similar changes were going on in other medical centers, like Johns Hopkins and the Columbia College of Physicians and Surgeons in New York. The Rockefeller Institute for Medical Research was founded in New York in 1902; its special hospital was opened in 1910. Francis Peabody had been one of the first Resident Physicians to work in this hospital, and his associates there knew all about the new development — they, too, were leaders in it. Evidently the change was general and not merely local. It stemmed from the Flexner Report.[1]

When the American Medical Association was reorganized in

1902 to become really representative of the profession through its House of Delegates and its Board of Trustees, one of its first achievements was the appointment of a Committee on Education.

It is hard to realize now that up to about 1910 there were many medical schools in this country which were run for the financial profit of their faculties, with little regard to any responsibility for the production of competent doctors. When the Education Committee of the American Medical Association, under Dr. Arthur Dean Bevan as Chairman and Dr. N. P. Colwell as Secretary, visited a number of these medical colleges, they found a shocking deficiency of teaching facilities. The Committee consulted with Mr. Henry S. Pritchett, President, and Mr. Abraham Flexner, member, of the Carnegie Foundation for the Advancement of Teaching, to see what to do about it, and the upshot was that Dr. Colwell and Mr. Flexner made a comprehensive survey of most of the schools. In 1910 their results were published in a document of 300-odd pages, which came to be known as the Flexner Report.

This report laid stress on the overproduction of uneducated, poorly trained medical practitioners, and it emphasized the need for proper facilities, especially laboratories, if education in medicine was to be adequate. It made this point among others: "A hospital under complete educational control is as necessary to a medical school as is a laboratory of chemistry or pathology." As might be expected, the Report excited much controversy, and, also as expected, it put many of the medical colleges out of business. It was responsible in part — indirectly perhaps — for bringing Dr. Edsall to Boston. The old order, in which promotions in the hospital and in the school depended largely on seniority, was coming to an end; the new order said that the Chief must be the best-qualified man obtainable from anywhere and that he must have the facilities and the opportunities to direct and share in the investigation of disease in medical research. The Flexner Report was the beginning of a new era in medicine.

When George came back from Baltimore, he was given a Dalton Scholarship to continue his work on blood. The first step was to find a place to work, and on looking around the Hospital he spied a small room next to the new chemical laboratory. The fact that Dr.

Denis had used the room to board a full-sized pig, so as to have fresh pig blood available at all times, was not appreciated at the moment. The room smelled of pig a little, but the stench was not too bad, and it was a wholesome rural sort of smell anyway. George saw that there was a good bench in front of the window where the north light was fine for work with the microscope. More important, he noted that the chemistry laboratory itself was next to the inner sanctum of Dr. J. Homer Wright, his old instructor-friend.

During the spring and summer of 1915, George worked in the little room, studying the patients with blood disorders. He saw again the variations in the shape and size and staining reactions of the blood cells, and he talked with Dr. Wright about his theories that some of the cells were young and immature, while others were old and well developed. The theories applied to the white cells — the leucocytes — quite as much as to the red cells.

All this time he was studying the dietary histories of the patients, for he was beginning to see that the diet had played an essential part in the cause of trouble. The young woman with hypochromic (pale blood) anemia and a lack of acid in her stomach was virtually cured when she was finally persuaded to eat a proper diet with plenty of meat and extra iron. Pellagra, sprue, beriberi, and pernicious anemia were diseases that had many symptoms in common. When patients with the first three of these were made to eat adequately, they all did well. Patients with pernicious anemia, however, did not respond so easily, and their blood smears were different. The red cells were large and well stained on the whole, but the smear showed variations in size and shape, and to find intact nuclei in some of them and the remains of nuclei in others suggested that these were young cells. The cells with intact nuclei are called blasts — normoblast or megaloblast depending on the size of the nucleus. In other cells, the small red spot is a Howell-Jolly body — the remains of the nucleus — and cells containing "jollies" are a trifle more mature than the blast cell. That idea led to the thought that the bone marrow was pushing its cells "off the assembly line" before construction was quite complete. When these findings were put together, the idea came that in pernicious anemia there might be some particular food substance which had a direct effect upon the growth of cells. George showed the smears to a girl who was learning to be a medical technician under Dr. Denis and told her: "The cell you have there is immature. When cells like that get out into the peripheral blood, it shows that the bone marrow is working too fast. If you find any more, let me see them." She remembers the episode to this day; George's enthusiasm was contagious.

Palmer and Gamble, Means, White, and Minot were the very first to enjoy the new regime, to profit by the progressive, aggressive, and inquisitive mind of Dr. Edsall. The difficulties under which they began their work are hard to comprehend. With their test tubes and burettes, their gasometers, galvanometers, and microscopes, they were pioneers quite as much as were Lewis and Clark with their caravans. Since that time, forty years ago, the progress in medicine is amazing. In May 1952, a seven-story Research Building, costing over $2,000,000, erected on the grounds of the Massachusetts General Hospital, was opened and dedicated. It contains nothing but laboratories, except for one or two library-classrooms and one or two offices for the heads of sections. In this building, doctors — a few Ph.D.'s as well as the M.D.'s — with technicians and secretaries, all work on a full-time basis, supported by grants of money contributed mostly for special purposes: "For the Study of Cancer," "For Heart Disease," "For an Electron Microscope," or "For the Use of Isotopes." When the Interurban Club meets today at the Massachusetts General Hospital, there is no difficulty in finding able young men to describe work that will appeal to anyone who wants to listen, almost regardless of his field of interest.

At home, in 1915, George and Marian were fixing their apartment, and they were quite "social," dining out with friends or having friends in to dine with them. Life was full and interesting. On Friday, August 27, 1915, "Dr. and Mrs." Minot came to Chappaquiddick to spend the week end with my mother and father. It was their first trip after their honeymoon, and they were both in good form, cheerful and happy; George looked better than I had seen him in some time. Marian was introduced to the good ship *Carryall*, and we sailed to the South Beach for afternoon tea. George was a little disturbed when my mother waded ashore, shoes and all, for he couldn't possibly get his feet wet, but otherwise he approved of everything. The kettle was boiled over a little fire of driftwood laid in a hole in the sand. My mother produced the sugar and cream, the bread and butter, as well as the tea, from her basket. She loved to have what she called her "P.M.T." on the beach. It was lovely sailing back, with the southwest breeze reduced to a gentle air, and the brilliant sunset on our weather beam.

That evening, George talked about the laboratory, about his interesting cases, and about his plans for practice in case he had any extra time in which to see private patients — and of course we talked about the war. We were upset by the loss of one or two of our friends, as well as the accounts we heard of experiences in the trenches and in the North Atlantic.

In September, Harvard College was beginning its new year, and Dr. Roger I. Lee, who was now in charge of student health, asked George to help him with the routine physical examinations of the incoming freshmen. To make careful examinations of nearly a thousand young men, and to do it in a short time, was a considerable business, and George and several other young doctors were quite active in Cambridge for a month or two. George did this work again during the next two years.

George was always busy. Our friend, Dr. Orville Rogers, who was House Physician at the M.G.H. in 1915, remembers seeing him "constantly bending over a microscope studying blood smears hour after hour." And Rogers adds, "He used to show me cells, which to his eye, better than to mine, deviated from the normal. I cannot remember any great light bursting on me, perhaps because it had not burst on George, but he was stringing the wires that later made the illumination possible." [2]

Dr. William J. Kerr writes:

> When I was a "striker" at the M.G.H., George Minot was one of my early inspirations. He and O. H. Robertson had a string of ten or fifteen patients with pernicious anemia on the wards all the time, and each one had to have complete blood counts and reticulocyte counts daily. Sometimes after splenectomy, when the cells were doing some fancy twists, there had to be even more frequent counts. At the time, I was a bit overwhelmed by the schedule, but I came to admire and respect the persistence and the capacity of those two fine men.[3]

It was Dr. Wright of the Pathology Laboratory who told George about the new stain called brilliant cresyl blue. This was a vital dye, so called because it could stain living cells without injuring them. When fresh blood was mixed with a solution of this brilliant cresyl blue, one could see small irregular lines running across certain of the red cells, which marked them as very young cells, released from the bone marrow a little before their full maturity. To discover the true significance of these marked cells, called reticulocytes, was a very important contribution. It was George who discovered that the percentage of reticulocytes in the peripheral blood gives a good index of bone-marrow activity. One of his notebooks shows interesting studies of reticulocytes, with many drawings of the cells in different cases. He was looking for some relation between the various forms that the markings in these curious cells displayed. It must have taken time to make the study of each case: "Patient W. on East Medical Service has Family Jaundice. The retics are 7.5% — definitely of the knotted type with good regular ones quite often. Not a few appear as very small jollies."

Dr. William Branch Porter, now Professor of Medicine at the Medical College of Virgina, remembers the several months that he spent in postgraduate study in Boston. Dr. Joseph H. Pratt had told him, "There is a young man at the Massachusetts General who will wake you up." George put Porter to work on reticulocytes, and when Porter left Boston George gave him a generous quantity of the brilliant cresyl blue dye in powder form. When the war came and the supply of German dye stopped, George offered Bill Porter a hundred dollars for the sample which he had given him. "The German dye is much better than we can make here," George wrote him.

In the meantime, George was working on two other projects. One was to observe the effect of acid on antithrombin. The other was to inject rabbits with hemoglobin — a gram of the "flakes" dissolved in 35 cc. of water — to see if hemoglobinuria, resulting in a red color to the urine, could be produced. It could not.

The transfusion of blood as an important treatment for hemorrhage, as well as for patients with severe anemia, was just beginning to be used. George, being the expert on blood, soon became the authority on transfusions. Shortly after his return from Baltimore, he wrote a very comprehensive paper[4] in which he reviewed recent work on the blood groups and the practical methods for determining

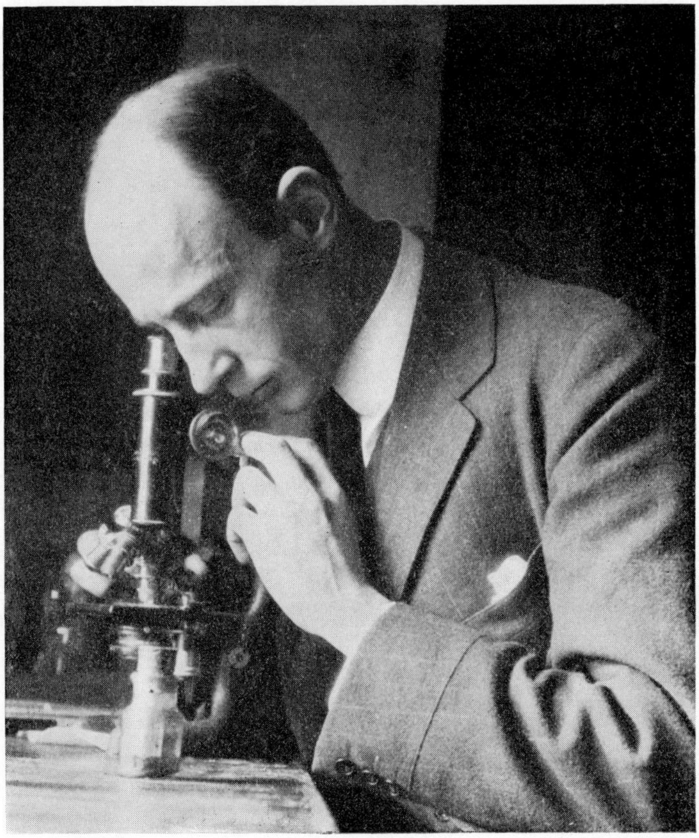

(*Photograph by Miss Catharine Thacher, 1917*)

THE INQUISITIVE PHYSICIAN

to which group the patient belonged, and so for selecting a donor whose blood would be suitable for that individual. With the help of two volunteers, Miss Margaret Weld, his wife's sister, and Miss Dorothy Mandell, who later became my wife, he collected a list of professional blood donors who were ready to be called to the hospital when blood of their particular groups was needed.

In those days, reactions after transfusions were not uncommon, in spite of the best technique for making sure that the patient and the donor belonged to the same blood group and that their two bloods were compatible with one another. George told the story of his visit to another hospital, where the worker on blood assured him: "No, Dr. Minot, we have no trouble with reactions so far as I know."

George asked him, "How many transfusions were made today?"

"We did five this morning."

"May I see the five patients? I am always interested in looking at patients an hour or two after they have had their transfusions."

When he arrived on the ward, there was considerable activity; the nurses were fetching new blankets and hot-water bottles, for each of the five patients was miserable with chills and fever — with reactions of greater or less severity. The doctor in charge was chagrined about this, for it became obvious that he had never taken the trouble to see what had happened to his patients after the procedure of transfusion had been finished.

During the winter of 1915–16 there was little change in the routine, but George had a number of irons in the fire. One was research with Dr. Roger I. Lee, whom George had helped with the student physical examinations at Harvard in September. Besides being in charge of student health at Harvard, Dr. Lee was Clinical Professor of Medicine in the Harvard Medical School, and Head of the West Medical Service at the Massachusetts General Hospital, opposite to Dr. Edsall on the East. Dr. Lee was very helpful and sympathetic to all the young men, and he and George developed a close relationship. Dr. Lee was also interested in the blood. He recognized George's ability and intelligence, and his chief interest was in helping the young man as much as possible. In that year George published "Studies on a Case of Idiopathic Purpura Hemorrhagica,"[5] and then later, with Dr. Lee and Dr. Beth Vincent, the surgeon, he published "Observations on Splenectomy in Pernicious Anemia. Studies on Bone Marrow Stimulation." [6]

There had been fifteen patients with pernicious anemia who had been treated by splenectomy as a possible life-saving measure. Three had died soon after operation, but in the other twelve George was delighted to observe that after the operation there was a marked increase in the number of reticulated red cells in the blood smear. Howell-Jolly bodies were also observed, and George recognized that young cells were being released from the bone marrow before they were quite ready. It was evident that the operation had produced a strong stimulation of the bone marrow. The difficulty, of course, was that there was only one spleen to be removed — only this one ace card to be played in the game. Although George's paper about his cases includes the statement that the reticulated red blood cells constitute a measure of bone-marrow activity, it is doubtful whether in that early day he had any idea of what these observations would later lead to. The study, however, had a further implication because it showed that it was possible to compare the blood picture after splenectomy with the blood picture observed in other cases where symptoms had subsided in a spontaneous remission. When the reticulocyte count went up, George recognized that spontaneous remissions had also depended on a stimulation of the bone marrow by some cause not yet known.

In May 1916, Drs. Roger I. Lee and George R. Minot gave their paper on the "Blood Platelets in Hemophilia" [7] before the meeting of the Association of American Physicians in Washington. They had observed that if normal blood platelets are added to hemophilic blood plasma, coagulation takes place normally, but when hemophilic platelets are added even in excess to normal plasma, the coagulation is delayed. The experimental results looked good, but as Dr. Castle[8] explained many years later, it was the technical difficulties of separating platelets unchanged and free of their "native" plasma that led Lee and Minot to the erroneous conclusion that the platelets in hemophilia were defective. We know today that the trouble is in the plasma protein.

In the summer of 1916, George and Marian took over the little cottage that their friend, Dr. Edward Reynolds, had built on the western shore of Vinal Haven Island, Maine. The cottage was a small frame house with four rooms, and George and Marian passed a very happy month there. They invited me to spend a few days of it with them. In their small boat it was easy to sail past the Sugar Loaves into North Haven, and also to sail in the other direction, through Ledbetter's Narrows, to explore the surrounding islands. It was beautiful country, and both George and Marian loved it.

To land on a strange island with George was always great fun, and it was instructive, too. He and Marian enjoyed the wild flowers, and they could name almost all of them. George saw the different varieties of spruce and cedar trees, and he would pick small samples to compare them directly. And then suddenly he would say, "Look at the blueberries over there! Let's get some," or "I bet we will find mountain cranberries just below that big rock up above." At noontime we would sit on some lovely spot, enjoy a good lunch, and then we would pick more blueberries in the afternoon. It was a very pleasant life.

In the fall of 1916 a great physical change took place at the Massachusetts General Hospital. The Moseley Building was opened, and the old M.G.H. lost something of its quaint simplicity. The House Pupils' Flat was no more, and all the young doctors were moved up to the new apartments on the third and fourth stories of this new building. The place was modern; the rooms were of fair size; there was even a pool table in one room, with a piano and a fireplace in another. The bathroom had showers as well as tubs. It was all very efficient and the new men might call it attractive, but for us the charm and the flavor of the old Flat had gone.

More important, the "Front Door" of the Hospital, with the administrative offices, was moved from the east end of the Bulfinch Building on Blossom Street to this new Moseley Building at the end of North Grove Street. Dr. Edsall was delighted to see the vacated space in the Bulfinch, and he lost no time in taking it over. All that space could now be used for research, and very soon Minot, Means, Rackemann, and Joseph C. Aub were each assigned to one of the rooms. This was a great improvement, and when Dr. Edsall found the money for equipment, the prospect of working in the new laboratories became quite exciting.

In January 1917, my diary notes: "G.R.M. and I spend money for the hospital." I can recall three or four large catalogues, with pictures of every kind of glassware, as well as of instruments and equipment in wide variety. We bought test tubes, pipettes, flasks, beakers, and petri dishes, all of assorted sizes; an incubator run by gas, a water bath, an autoclave, and a "hot box," or oven, in which to sterilize glassware; a centrifuge and a good-sized icebox. We had a field day with the catalogue, and we were quite delighted when Dr. Edsall approved of almost everything in the long list that we had compiled.

The boxes and the barrels did not arrive until that summer, but I remember the excitement when they finally came, and the busyness of moving all of our equipment from the old Chem Lab and setting up modern laboratories in the new space provided by the wisdom of Dr. Edsall.

On April 28, 1917, the same day that President Wilson signed the Draft Law, I was married to Dorothy Mandell. George was best man for me, as I had been for him. Both George and I drew high numbers in the draft, so there was no great hurry to decide what we had better do.

At the Massachusetts General Hospital, the Superintendent, Doctor (or rather Colonel) Frederick A. Washburn, was rushing through his plans to organize the M.G.H. Unit — Base Hospital No. 6. On May 24, Dr. Paul D. White was ordered to active duty to enlist the noncommissioned personnel. On July 9, with great secrecy, Base Hospital No. 6 left Boston, and on July 11 the *Aurania* carried the 26 medical officers, 66 nurses, and 155 corpsmen out of New York Harbor. They left a large hole behind them.

If life at home had been busy before, the pressure of work after the Unit left was terrific. George had been appointed Assistant in Medicine to the Harvard Medical School, and he had to talk to students and arrange the details of their work. He had his laboratory to keep alive, and he had to be ready for special work on blood problems. Besides this, he had patients to see in the outpatient clinic, on the wards, and in his private office. He was on the run about fifteen hours a day.

On Monday, July 30, a new group of Fourth-Year students arrived at the M.G.H. The school had been put on an accelerated program, which cut out most of the summer free time, and provided three terms instead of two for each calendar year. George was the instructor in charge of the M.G.H. course in medicine, and on the first day he gave the students a long talk. They must learn to take good histories, make physical examinations that were careful and complete, and be keen observers and good recorders of what they saw. It was his first responsible teaching assignment.

In August and September 1917, George was employed for a short time as a Contract Surgeon in the Army, and was sent to the various Army camps in New England to examine the recruits of the Twenty-sixth Division for tuberculosis and heart disease. The recruits bored him excessively. He did not care for any work that was pure routine, and the business of examining young men, "thousands of them," one after another as they filed past in a line for four tedious hours every morning appealed to him not at all. There was no challenge to his thinking powers, only the "stupid routine," necessary though it might be. However, he hung on through August and most of September.

During the fall and winter of 1917–18, George worked hard in the new laboratory. In addition to the large amount of routine work, he found time in 1917 to publish seven papers, four of them on the blood platelets. He brought together the scattered knowledge about their nature and origin, and he discussed their significance in disease. Other work improved his own understanding of the bone marrow and its functions. The bone marrow makes all the different kinds of blood cells — the red cells as well as the white cells and the platelets. Disorders of the bone marrow can result in the faulty production of one kind of cells, or of all the cells at once. For example, in the disease called purpura hemorrhagica, the small black-and-blue spots on the skin are the result of tiny hemorrhages which are caused sometimes by a lack of blood platelets. In agranulocytosis, only the granular cells — the polymorphs — are involved, but in aplastic anemia the bone marrow loses all of its function and all of the blood cells, both white and red, are deficient at the same time. Needless to say, this last is a very serious condition. In one paper[9] George pointed out that each of these conditions depends upon a poison — a toxin of some sort — that has injured the bone marrow in one or all of its functional parts.

In his paper, written with Dr. J. Homer Wright, on "The Viscous Metamorphosis of the Blood Platelets,"[10] he showed the several circumstances under which the platelets seemed to agglutinate in masses and strands to play their role in the clotting process.

Here is a typical item in his notebooks:

> May 15. Patient . . . is better this week. Platelets strike the eye as fully normal size. Many are large: some huge. Angular, boomerang, elongated shapes. Oval, round, often coarse looking — plain with a few dots. Some are queer: very dark in the center. Some small also to be sure, but the character is clearly abnormal. All kinds of curious platelets.

As one reads these notes, one gains the impression that his mind was working about three jumps ahead of his pencil. There was no thought about the form of notes; all he wanted was to get every detail recorded. Even the slightest variations were put down in his notebook.

During this time the office at 188 Marlborough Street was rapidly becoming George's office. A few private patients were referred to him for consultations, and that was an added responsibility. Dr. Edsall would caution him: "Go at it slowly. Don't try to do it all at once." It was good advice. George engaged a secretary, Miss Marjorie Curtis, who was tolerant of his many idiosyncrasies. His dictation was terrible — hesitating and full of changes — and when it came to the unscrambling of his handwriting, it took imagination and experience to translate it. Besides, this writing was on bits of paper, any old paper. The back of an envelope or advertisement, or often a postcard, might bear a message of considerable value. George never learned how to fold a letter. He never could fold the paper in threes; quarters did not fit the envelope, and the edge had to be given an extra fold to jam it in. Never mind! The finished product was always interesting and worth having.

In September, he and Marian had moved from the apartment to a house at 247 Beacon Street, around the corner from 188 Marlborough Street. They had more space for work and entertainment; they were more independent.

During all of 1918, the routine was terrific. George was "hopelessly busy," as he would say. So many doctors were away that those of us still at home were hard pressed to keep up with the work. George was teaching on the medical wards and in the Out-Patient Department at the M.G.H. In March, the Faculty of Harvard Medical School made him Assistant Professor of Medicine, and he began to take an active part in the curriculum. A course of lectures to the Third Year students was arranged. There was little time for any investigative work in the laboratory.

That summer there was trouble in one of the munitions factories in New Jersey. Workers were being poisoned by contact with a chemical of some sort. Weakness and debility, sometimes actual prostration, were the symptoms, and anemia, resulting from injury to the bone marrow, was the diagnosis. Dr. Alice Hamilton[11] had done excellent work in the new field of industrial medicine, describing the lesions and the diseases produced by exposure to the dusts and the fumes of heavy metals, as well as to many organic compounds, especially the derivatives of benzol. She had worked at the Massachusetts General Hospital from time to time under the aegis of Dr. Edsall. George Minot always admired her knowledge, as well as her way of approaching complex problems, and she in turn admired him, having recognized his "infinite capacity for taking pains." It was through Dr. Hamilton that the Army appointed George Minot again as a Contract Surgeon, this time as an expert to investigate the trouble in the New Jersey munitions factories. George spent several weeks examining the victims and making meticulous studies of their blood pictures. This army job was a challenge to his thinking powers, and he enjoyed it.

"Blood Examinations of Trinitrotoluene Workers" was the title of a paper[12] that he published in 1919. In this careful and comprehensive study, George presented the evidence for excessive red blood cell destruction by the poison chemical, and the evidence of increased blood formation, nature's effort to repair the damage. He showed that, in the majority of the victims, the effect of the poison was temporary, and therefore the process was reversible. In case, however, exposure to the poison went beyond a certain point the excessive blood destruction might produce a toxic hemolytic jaundice, and the resulting anemia might be fatal. A little later came another project: to find the nature of the trouble from ether in the manufacture of smokeless powder. Dr. Hamilton and George wrote a paper[13] describing their observations.

Meantime, my own orders had come in March to report to the Commanding Officer of the Base Hospital at Camp Merritt, New Jersey. Later, Dorothy and I were delighted to find that the house in which we lived in Englewood, New Jersey, was not far from the munitions factory, and that George could stay with us. It was good to have him, and, as always, his talk was stimulating. He reviewed and explained some of his own findings, and then he asked questions about my work. I had to explain that the Base Hospital at Camp Merritt was not like the M.G.H., and that we did the routine as well as we could and let it go at that!

In September 1918, a dreadful plague struck America. It struck Europe, too. The influenza epidemic was catastrophic. It happened that the Base Hospital at Camp Merritt was being enlarged, and several new pavilion wards were almost ready for occupancy. I remember the trainload of farmer boys from the "cotton and corn" region, who arrived sick. We put them to bed in new wards as soon as we could, and they lay there motionless, soundless, prostrate. Next morning they were still prostrate, but on the third morning a few would turn their heads to see who was coming into the ward. On the fourth morning most of the men were sitting up, but one or two were still prostrate. When we listened to the lungs of these two, pneumonia was well defined. Then the sick ones from all over the hospital were assembled in a special ward, where many of them — in fact, most of them — died. It was a ghastly, horrible business, all the more so because there was so little that we could do about it. If only we had had penicillin in those days!

George was back at Boston at that time. He himself escaped the infection, and Marian escaped, too, except for a mild illness in February 1919. This was extra fortunate, because her baby was due to arrive in the fall, and it had been found in most cases that pregnancy lowered the patient's resistance. Needless to say, George and Cousin Jim were worried about her. A few days later, their maid fell ill, and she was moved to the M.G.H., where the disease advanced to fulminating proportions, and where three days later she died. Marian's escape was appreciated all the more.

On October 6, 1918, little Marian Linzee Minot was born quite safely at 247 Beacon Street. George was delighted to be relieved of a heavy anxiety, and he was almost as pleased as Marian was to have a daughter.

Harvard College opened again on September 23, in the midst of the epidemic. Dr. Roger I. Lee was Counsultant in Medicine to the 3d Army Corps, A.E.F., but once more George was working with the Harvard Hygiene Department, this time, however, as part of the Army. His duty was to supervise the physical examinations of candidates for the Harvard Student Army Training Corps. Others were there, too, including Dr. Robert F. Loeb, who today is Chief of Medicine at the Presbyterian Hospital in New York. President Lowell had organized the college on a military basis; the Student Army Training Corps was divided into companies and then regiments, about 1500 men each. Fourth Year medical students were assigned as Company "Doctors." The program of routine physical examinations was accelerated, and when any man was found to have a fever, he was sent to the hospital immediately. All students who lived at home were requested, and later ordered, to stay at college — for the first three days in a quarantined dormitory — to keep out of contact with the general public. After September 30, all lectures and classes for over fifty men were stopped; indeed, between September 30 and October 21 the whole teaching program was brought almost to a standstill. Later, George and Dr. Loeb described in a formal paper the attempt to prevent influenza at Harvard.[14]

On November 11, 1918, the Armistice was signed by Marshal Foch and the Germans. The crowds of people singing and dancing in Times Square had their counterparts in Boston, but neither George nor Marian wore paper hats or blew on tin whistles on Tremont Street. Their reaction was less demonstrative.

For two years, George Minot worked on his problems in blood diseases at the Massachusetts General Hospital, and then he became more and more interested in the activities at the Collis P. Huntington Memorial Hospital, which had been open for five years and which was known as a "cancer hospital." There were several reasons for this new interest. The first is probably the most important: Dr. Francis W. Peabody, whom George had admired so much, was at that time Consulting Physician to the Huntington, in addition to his regular service as Associate Physician to the Peter Bent Brigham Hospital. Francis Peabody was a delightful person — gentle, dignified, tactful, and forceful when necessary — who was admired by everybody, and especially by George Minot. Francis Peabody knew much about disease, but he knew even more about patients, for he loved people.

He was a good Doctor, with a capital "D," and he was a good teacher, too. His lecture in the Sunday afternoon series at the Medical School on "The Care of the Patient" [15] is the oft-quoted medical classic, which ends with this sentence:

> One of the essential qualities of the clinician is interest in humanity, for the secret of the care *of* the patient is in caring *for* the patient.

When Francis Peabody suggested that George should join him at the Huntington, it was hard to refuse the opportunity that seemed to offer so much. The Huntington Hospital was a brand new place, unhampered by traditions, and the chance for a new approach to George's problems was a challenge that was exciting. George knew that the Huntington was a center for the study of leukemia, one of the important blood diseases. Leukemia is characterized by an enormous increase in the numbers of white cells, or leucocytes, in the tissues, and especially in the blood. The increase depends on an extensive proliferation or multiplication of one or several of the primitive stem cells from which leucocytes arise. The cells seen in the peripheral blood are young, immature cells, their types varying according to the particular stem cell from which they come.

It was easy to compare this excessive production to the overgrowth of other cells in tumors, and so it came about that leukemia was regarded as a tumor of the blood. If that were true, George realized that the study of leukemia might well be correlated with the study of other tumors and also with the study of anemia. New knowledge about leukemia, or about cancer, for that matter, might suggest some new approach to anemia, and conversely, what was learned about anemia might lead to new knowledge about cancer. The Huntington was obviously an excellent place in which to make comparative observations of this kind, and the more familiar George became with this hospital, the more he appreciated the opportunities that it presented.

The origin of the Cancer Commission of Harvard University is described in the First Annual Report of the Collis P. Huntington Memorial Hospital, for the year 1912. The pertinent section reads:

RESEARCH AT M.G.H. AND HUNTINGTON

In 1899, by the will of the late Caroline Brewer Croft, a sum of money was left in trust for the study of cancer. In 1901 additional funds became available, and the Cancer Commission of Harvard University was established by the President and Fellows of Harvard College. Some time later, the Commission realized that if patients with cancer were to be studied by systematic laboratory methods, hospital facilities would be needed, and so efforts were made to procure still more funds. Through the generous gift of Mrs. Collis P. Huntington, an amount sufficient to build the hospital was secured, and additional gifts provided a modest endowment fund in addition to the Caroline Brewer Croft Fund already available.[16]

The Cancer Commission was composed of six distinguished men: Dr. Henry K. Oliver and Dr. John Collins Warren to represent the Croft Fund; Dr. Henry P. Wolcott and Dr. Edward H. Bradford, Dean of the Medical School, to represent the Harvard Corporation; and Dr. William T. Councilman and Dr. Theobald Smith to represent the Medical School. Dr. Ernest E. Tyzzer was Director of the Commission, Dr. Robert B. Greenough was Secretary, and Mr. Arthur Adams was Treasurer.

This hospital was not designed as a place for the custodial care of chronic invalids. On the contrary, it was to be, in essence, a laboratory, a workshop, where patients with malignant disease could be studied from many points of view, and where various methods of treatment could be applied and, if successful, perhaps the mechanism of their effect might be evaluated and so lead to new studies and new approaches to the cancer problem. In the summer of 1912, the year of George's graduation from medical school, the Collis P. Huntington Memorial Hospital, built on Huntington Avenue in close proximity to Harvard Medical School, was opened. Many patients were sent in for consultation. The really sick ones were admitted to the small wards, but the majority were seen and followed from time to time by appointment in the outpatient department. The first staff of the Huntington was made up of eminent men, well qualified to start the work of the Hospital on a high plane of efficiency.

Dr. Tyzzer, Director of the Hospital, had been working on those problems in pathology that are concerned with the growth of tissues and cells. A very quiet, profound thinker, he had already established the first strains of mice with high tumor and low tumor incidence. Dr. Clarence C. Little, realizing the importance of this discovery, came to the Huntington to work with Dr. Tyzzer on this problem, and so established his life interest. Little's work in genetics, which had begun at Harvard under Dr. William E. Castle, was fostered at the Huntington; it continued when he was President of the University of Michigan, and it goes on today at the Roscoe B. Jackson Memorial Laboratory in Bar Harbor, Maine, where he is Director, and where there is a very important colony of mice, bred some for resistance and some for susceptibility to tumor transplants.

Dr. William Duane was a physicist of considerable experience and renown. Deeply interested in x-ray therapy, and realizing the need for penetrating radiation, he developed a 200,000-volt x-ray machine at the Huntington. He and the clinicians did much to evaluate the effects of radium in cancer and to compare them with the effects of his high-voltage x-ray therapy. The high-voltage machine was found to have interesting effects on leukemia, and this offered a field of research that interested George Minot. It was Dr. Duane who defined the "r" (roentgen) unit as a measure of x-ray potency.

Dr. Ordway, the first Physician-in-Charge, was a capable practitioner with a broad mind and plenty of common sense. Dr. Henry A. Christian and Dr. Robert B. Greenough, who had been our teachers, were Consulting Physician and Consulting Surgeon, respectively.

Francis Peabody, Consulting Physician to the Huntington, had been interested in leukemia. When in May 1917 he went on a Red Cross mission to Rumania, his work was taken up by George Minot and Dr. Gerald Blake, an excellent practitioner who was soon to be associated with George in private practice. At first Jerry Blake and George worked at the Huntington on a volunteer basis, without any official appointment, but in 1918 George was made Assistant Consulting Physician, and so had authority in the Hospital. During the war, he and Dr. Blake could do little investigation; the routine clinical work was far too demanding.

In the spring of 1919, however, when Francis Peabody came back from his consulting service with the American Army in France, George was promoted to Physician, and he and Dr. Blake were authorized to go ahead with the leukemia problem, as well as with

George's own special study of the megakaryocytes in the blood in leukemia. Dr. Peabody helped George in this. A colored plate of the cells was prepared. Francis Peabody and George talked about writing a complete monograph on leukemia, but their work was never published in any such comprehensive form.

George had two excellent students working with him. Dr. Arthur H. Gundersen did further work with the blood platelets, counting their numbers in various stages of leukemia. Dr. Thomas E. Buckman worked on the chemical characteristics of the white blood cells. George wanted to clarify certain ideas about the relation between leukemia, with its excess of leucocytes in the blood, and polycythemia, with its excess of red cells. George and Tom Buckman worked together on leukemia for over two years, and their studies included the effect of treatment with x-ray at the M.G.H. and with radium at the Huntington, and a comparison of the two methods. George had a high regard for Tom Buckman. He recognized that his inquiring spirit gave great promise for his future. The news of Buckman's untimely death in 1945 came as a real shock to George.

While George and his students were working on the blood, Dr. Channing C. Simmons was working on the relation between Hodgkin's disease and lymphosarcoma. It is obvious that there were many different angles to the over-all problem.

At the weekly conferences, the progress of the different projects was discussed, and the plans for the next steps were outlined, and often modified. George was critical and practical; he maintained that in each case the object of the study, the question to be answered, must be kept clearly in mind, although sometimes it was important to follow a secondary lead that might be opened by the results of preliminary investigation. His advice was sound and helpful. He was injecting his young assistants with some of his own insatiable inquisitiveness.

All this time, George's work was attracting attention. Dr. Elliott P. Joslin, who had lectured to us on diabetes, had a well-to-do patient whose husband had pernicious anemia. They wanted advice about the treatment of the man's anemia, and Dr. Joslin sent them to George. In doing so, he suggested that if they would enable George to travel to New York and Baltimore to see what progress was being made in the study of blood disease in these centers, George might be able to make his advice about treatment even better. So soon as they saw George, they realized that Dr. Joslin's description of him as a "brilliant young investigator" fitted exactly. A little later they gave George a check for $1,000, and both George and Marian were highly gratified. Dr. Joslin was pleased too.

George's own move from the Massachusetts General Hospital to the Huntington had been made gradually: less and less work done in the old place, more and more in the new. There is no specific date for the transition.

Elizabeth Whitney Minot, George and Marian's second daughter, was born on December 4, 1920, at 247 Beacon Street. All had gone very well with mother and child, but this was another very pleasant interest and an added responsibility. Life was becoming more complex each day. Whenever my wife and I would dine at the Minots' house, or they would come to us, George would say, "Rack, I am tired," and would add, "I have had an awful day — forty-eleven things to do, and no chance to sit down. Goodness knows, I wish I were not so hopelessly busy, so that we could meet more often."

Both George and Marian realized the importance of outside interests to keep the horizon broad. Dining out to spend a pleasant evening with friends was one way of doing it. Another way was to invite friends to a dinner party, and Marian Minot was most skillful in arranging many delightful evenings at 247 Beacon Street. She knew whom George would like to see and talk with when the men were drinking their coffee and brandy after dinner. On Sunday nights, quite regularly, the three Minot brothers dined with their father at 188 Marlborough Street, and Marian went with George. The brothers were close to each other, and although George knew even less about the business world — both Jimmy and Henry held positions in the investment field — than they knew about medicine, nevertheless he was interested in hearing them talk about such mundane topics as stocks, bonds, and politics. Cousin Jim and Marian were interested, too, but for them George's many activities were much more exciting and more understandable. The talk before the fire in their father's library was usually good talk. One topic that interested the whole group was the problem of where one could find money to support medical research. As medical knowledge advanced, and the demand for laboratories and equipment increased, the question was becoming ever more important.

There were other activities that changed the scene and the pace. The Medical Exchange Club had its first meeting on May 13, 1920. Drs. E. Granville Crabtree, genitourinary surgeon, Elliott C. Cutler, general surgeon, George R. Minot, expert on blood, Francis M. Rackemann, interested in anaphylaxis and allergy, and Philip D. Wilson, orthopedic surgeon, agreed that it would be a fine idea if our "great minds," each centered on a different aspect of medicine or surgery, could meet once a month or so to have dinner together and to "exchange" our thoughts. No man can be entirely familiar with more than one field of medical science. Knowledge of his own subject may be complete from top to bottom — vertical knowledge — but in addition he needs to know something about certain levels in other subjects — horizontal knowledge. It is easy to overlook the fact that similar problems come up in other fields and that the specific information required in one field may apply to the others as well. Meantime, if the approach has been from a different angle, a new thought may result. There was every reason to hope that an informal exchange of ideas might be helpful to each of us. The continued success to this day of our Medical Exchange Club can be attributed to the fact that at each meeting there is "intellectual" as well as "gustatory pabulum," as Jim Gamble puts it. We enjoy our meetings all the more because we learn so much.

At the first meeting, Dr. James Howard Means, Dr. Cecil Kent Drinker, and Dr. Andrew Watson Sellards were elected to membership. The third meeting was held on October 15, 1920, with George as host at his father's house. After an excellent dinner, George prefaced his remarks with quotations from John Locke, James Jackson, and Henry I. Bowditch, each of whom had laid stress on the thorough examination of the patient as a whole. He went on to tell us about megakaryocytes and the occasional appearance of these cells in the peripheral blood, and then he discussed the various features that polycythemia, leukemia, and pernicious anemia have in common. Dr. Drinker remarked that this was not surprising, because all blood cells originate from a sort of primordial cell in the bone marrow. To this Cutler commented that a transmutation of cells like this is a little hard to contemplate. In tumors, the new cells differ from the original, but the change is in only one direction. To consider that a primordial cell in the marrow can give rise to a whole series of white cells on the one hand, and to a series of red blood cells on the other, is not easy. This repartee showed that the idea of exchanging our knowledge and ideas was developing profitably, as we had anticipated.

At the next few meetings, Dr. Ernest W. Goodpasture, expert on viruses, Dr. Stanley Cobb, neurologist, Dr. Frederick Carpenter Irving, obstetrician, Dr. James Lawder Gamble, pediatrician and chemist, Dr. Kenneth Daniel Blackfan, pediatrician, and Dr. Richard Henry Miller, general surgeon, each was elected unanimously.

There was another dining club to which George and I belonged. It was very different from the Medical Exchange Club. Soon after college, a group of men in the Harvard classes of 1908, 1909, and 1910 had organized the Planet Club — its name intended to indicate its "worldwide" interests — the prime movers in a group of about thirty men being Augustus Peabody Loring, Jr., and Edward Wigglesworth, George's Harvard College classmates. These meetings were good fun, of course, and through them we came to know more intimately those of our contemporaries who had become lawyers, bankers, merchants, and manufacturers, and whose interests were different from ours. The intellectual fare, however, was limited to the ribald stories which some of the members could tell with real artistry, to produce gales of laughter. The Planet Club faded out as we grew older because it had no fundamental purpose. Incidentally, George Minot never could tell a story. If he happened to think of the "motif," he could not remember how it began, and if he did remember the first part, he could not bring out the point.

In 1920, George Minot was made President of the Boylston Medical Society. Each year, the Third Year students who were members of the "Boylston" chose a member of the faculty to preside over their weekly meetings, at which only this one older man was present. George recognized that it was a great compliment to be chosen, and he accepted the honor, knowing full well what the devotion of one night every week would do to his work program. For his presidential speech, George gave "A Rambling Address on Medical Science and Art," which began this way: "In 1846 — seventy-five years ago —

Henry J. Bigelow was President of your Society, and his Address was entitled, 'Fragments of Medical Science and Art.' " George's notes, on nine pages of yellow paper, are still in his file. They show that he talked about types of practice, commercialism, and fees, about the importance of careful notes, and of time to meditate: "The only time that serious errors are excusable is when the need for haste is conspicuous." Then he added his favorite theme: "Try to think of the patient as a whole person — a knowledge of human nature and of different personalities is important, and this requires that the doctor know something about worldly affairs, and that he learn to keep his field of vision broad." George's talks to students, no matter how informal, were prepared carefully; the best that he could do in the choice of topics and the choice of words was none too good for the students.

During the war, George began to give lectures to the Third Year, and later to the Second Year, students. He and Dr. James Howard Means developed a course of lectures on applied physiology that was designed to integrate preclinical science with clinical medicine — with the talks that Dr. William H. Robey and Dr. Cyrus C. Sturgis were giving to the student sections in the hospitals. A few sentences taken from the notes for introduction show how mature were George's thoughts:

The "Theory and Practice of Physic" is a good designation for this part of your course in Medicine. Anyone taking care of the sick must be a physician. Knowledge of pathology is essential, and it includes a knowledge of anatomy — the structure of the body — and a knowledge of physiology — the functions of the different parts and tissues of the body. Our aims are the prevention of disease — the early diagnosis of all those disorders which lead to serious difficulties later on. Success in diagnosis will come to him who sees the whole course of his case. The progress of medicine will be hampered and delayed until the practitioner becomes an investigator. Every case presents a problem which must be solved. The ability to use your eyes and ears and hands — all your senses — to gather information, and the development of your thinking power to interpret that information, is what we must teach you. Mechanical machines, like the x-ray, and all the methods of the laboratory, will help you, but they, too, must be interpreted. Special lectures or short courses in one disease are not designed to train you as specialists — but rather to teach you which patients require specialized examinations. The results of treatment are often very difficult to evaluate — and for many reasons. One of them is the overenthusiasm of the doctor — particularly of the so-called specialist: the other is the modern tendency to forget the value of the simplest clinical methods — a complete and careful history and a complete and careful physical examination, with attention to the patient as a whole human being. Clinical vision should be sharpened and not dulled by the light of science. An inquisitive spirit is to be cultivated: imagination is an important part of it, but the conclusions must be subjected to adequate test and critical control.

In September 1921, Francis Peabody resigned as Consulting Physician and Chief of the Medical Service at the Huntington Hospital in order to become Director of the new Thorndike Memorial Laboratory at the Boston City Hospital. This was a blow to the Huntington, but the members of the Cancer Commission had no great difficulty in deciding that the man to be appointed as Peabody's successor was George R. Minot. George was now in the full swing of his work, and he was well qualified to take over the organization of the medical service and its laboratories. The appointment caused some excitement in the Minot family, but, after all, it was not a tremendous surprise. There is a photograph that shows George Minot and Francis Peabody sitting on the piazza at Northeast Harbor engaged in serious conversation, and it is fair to assume that they were talking about Peabody's new job at the Thorndike and about his successor at the Huntington.

"Rack," George said to me later, "did you hear that I am to have a new job? Francis Peabody says he thinks I can do it all right. Do you suppose my health and strength are good enough to stand the strain?"

"Of course you can do it!" I said. "I congratulate you, and I congratulate the Huntington, too."

George was a young man of only thirty-five years, but he was good enough to be put in charge of an important unit. His approach to the new job is shown by the notes for the introduction to one of his Third Year lectures:

> A man with no imagination may collect facts, but he cannot make great discoveries. Claude Bernard used to say, "When you enter the laboratory put off your imagination as you take off your overcoat, but so soon as you leave, put it on again."
>
> When we have all the facts that science can discover, we need often not only scientific interpretation, but also a spiritual interpretation. The

power of transforming facts so that they become facts plus interpretation is one of the most distinctive elements in human life. Happiness is not an outward event, but an inward interpretation. Facts alone are like pieces of irritating grit that get into the oyster shell; it is through interpretation of them that the pearl of life is created. Progress should be orderly and stable. Morgagni was interested in organs, Bichat in tissues, but Virchow thought about cells, and nowadays we approach the fluids within and between the cells.

George took over the direction of the medical service at the Huntington in September 1921. It was only about a month later that the course of his life took a sudden and serious turn.

7

Diabetes

At noon on October 12, 1921, George's brother Jimmy (James Jackson Minot, Jr.) was married to Miss Miriam Sears at St. John's Church in Pride's Crossing, Beverly, Massachusetts. The day was cold, raw, and rainy, with thunder showers. That morning, George and Marian drove down to Beverly with Jimmy, Henry, and his father. Henry was to be Jimmy's best man, and George was to be an usher. George was not well on that morning. He felt bad, and he looked bad; he said he felt very tired and weak. He had felt tired before, but this time the reason did not seem obvious. Then he realized quite suddenly that he had been thirsty more than before and had been drinking water in quantity. Just to play safe, he later tested his own urine for sugar, and on the next day he telephoned me in the late afternoon.

"Rack, can you come over here pretty soon? I'm in trouble. I'd be glad if you could come right away."

I dropped everything, of course, and almost ran to 247 Beacon Street. George looked about the same as usual, but it was obvious that he and Marian were worried and frightened about something.

"What's the trouble?" I said.

His reply was slow and deliberate. "Sugar was found in my urine today, and there is quite a lot of it. It looks as though I have diabetes. You know what that means. With my poor health and thin body, it may be serious. Here I am in the middle of a lot of things that interest me greatly, and I would be very unhappy if I had to give up at this point."

"You feel all right in general, don't you?" I asked.

"Sure! The fact is that I have felt better than usual this summer; that is, up until the last month. It is very disturbing, and whatever happens it is going to be pretty hard on Marian. What do you think?"

"Well," I said, "the first thing to do is to find out exactly what this is all about. Is it really diabetes? And if so, how bad is it?"

"That's right," he said. "When we get some facts, we can go on from there."

"The first thing to do is to see Dr. Joslin," I put in.

"Yes, of course," George said, and Marian added, "We have already telephoned him, and we're going to see him tomorrow."

Dr. Elliott P. Joslin was, and still is, the highest authority on diabetes, not only in this country, but in the world. He had lectured to our class in the Medical School, and his textbook on diabetes is still a standard reference.[1] Equally important now, he was a friend whom George — and I too — admired and respected greatly.

If the finding of sugar in the urine was confirmed, and especially if the blood contained an abnormal quantity of sugar (glucose), the diagnosis of diabetes would be established, and the matter was serious. There was no insulin in those days, and diabetes could be a dangerous malady, as both George and I knew. At that first moment, it was hard for me to know what to say or do, except to cheer George and Marian on as best I could. I learned that the urine had been examined six months before this, in March 1921, and found to be clear. One can imagine what a shock this new finding must have been to George's father, so devoted to his boys and so very proud of what George had accomplished.

The record of George Minot's case (No. 2383), which Dr. Joslin still holds in his file, is a remarkable collection of data, with letters and notes of many kinds added in. It begins with George's first visit, on Saturday, October 15, 1921. George was not quite thirty-six years old. Sugar in the urine amounted to 7.1 grams per 100 cubic centimeters. Sugar in the blood was up to 430 milligrams per 100 cubic centimeters (percent), the normal being around 100 milligrams. George weighed only 135 pounds, which meant that this man, who was 6 feet 1½ inches tall, was very thin. The weight loss, however, had not been great. He had never weighed more than 147 pounds; he reached this maximum in 1912 while in medical school. In November 1920, one year before the discovery of diabetes, his weight was down to 142 pounds.

On the evening of this first visit to Dr. Joslin, my wife and I went down to 247 Beacon Street again.

"How did you get along?" I asked.

"Dr. Joslin was very kind to us. He told us that the road ahead is hard and long, but that he had other patients like me. It was interesting to have him talk to us in the way that he told us in his lecture to talk to our patients. You remember what he said about the management of patients? 'When they have understood the principles of the burning of sugar in the body, when they have learned to control themselves and to follow the diet without cheating, and when they have kept a daily record of food intake and sugar excretion to serve as a guide to treatment, they have come out all right.' He told us to expect trouble at first, but said that we would learn fast. We must be neither anxious nor afraid. Goodness knows it's lucky we have Dr. Joslin to go to. He told us that he had an increasing list of patients whose diabetes is severe, but who nevertheless have done very well."

"What are you going to do about the Huntington?" I asked.

"Dr. Joslin said that I not only *can* keep on, I have *got* to keep on. Hard work will not hurt me at all."

"That's wonderful!" I said. "Doesn't he want you to go to the hospital for a few days to be studied?"

"No, he said that since Marian and I had some idea about diabetes to start with, it was not necessary to instruct us in the basic principles — he could trust us to follow his directions without preliminary demonstrations."

"Well," I said, "aren't you even going to lay off for a few days?"

"Lay off? No! Why should I?" And then George added, "By the way, I would be very grateful if you would keep this business to yourselves. There is no use in having anyone know of my trouble, and all the more so if I do not have to stop my work on account of it. I am going to the Hospital just as usual."

And go he did. And on the next day, even though it was Sunday. As I write this account, Dr. Joslin wants me to "insert a fact — that he [George Minot] had so much backbone that following the detection of sugar, he did not let it break his routine even for a moment. He went *each* day to his work in the hospital, even on the *very next day.*" At the bottom of his note, Dr. Joslin adds appreciatively, "That blessed character!"

At a later visit, Dr. Joslin was thinking about the cause of George's disease. What about heredity? Was there anyone in the Minot family or the Whitney family who had had diabetes? No, George's father had good family records, and he could not find any evidence that George had inherited a taint that would have made him more predisposed to diabetes than the average person. Factors within George himself were considered. All his life there had been emphasis on food, and George had eaten well. In his childhood, he was always thin and delicate, and his father had encouraged him — sometimes almost forced him — to eat more than he wanted. Did these habits lead to a "strain" of any kind? It was hard to say.

George had suffered all his life from "stomach-aches," more than the rest of us. Sometimes the pains in his upper abdomen and across his lower back were quite severe. However, they did not interfere with his activities; the "aches" seemed to pass off in minutes rather than in hours. They were like a cramp of some kind. Dr. Joslin thought about disturbances of the pancreas, but there was no good way of ruling the idea either in or out.

Dr. Joslin laid some stress on the fact that George had had a good vacation during the previous summer. He and Marian, with little Marian, aged almost three, and the baby, Elizabeth, aged seven months, had rented a cottage at Pocasset on Cape Cod. It was a perfect place for the children, and to have a good nurse to take care of them made it easy for George and Marian to be off for the day with a picnic lunch, to "inspect" various parts of the surrounding country. For them, the Cape was not so attractive as the coast of Maine, but the summer there made an interesting change. However, George had not felt well. His indigestion was troublesome.

Marian had taken her excellent cook and her parlormaid to Pocasset, and the food was wonderful. During the vacation, George had hoped to gain weight. He ate extra crackers, and butter, and chocolate, for he seemed to be always hungry. In spite of his eating and resting, however, his weight stayed the same.

In September he had been extremely busy, but, even so, he felt less tired than in the spring. It is true that two weeks before the onset, he had caught a cold, but he felt poorly for only forty-eight hours. In retrospect, it is tempting to believe that this infection, although quite mild, had been the last straw in precipitating the disease.

At the first visit to Dr. Joslin, a daily diet of 189 grams of carbohydrate, 89 grams of protein, and 15 grams of fat was prescribed. George and Marian were told that from now on every morsel of food that he put into his mouth must be weighed or measured, and recorded accurately. Scales, with pad and pencil, were to become a necessary encumbrance to the table at every meal. The composition of all the different foods must be learned thoroughly so that the daily intake would be known exactly.

"The record of food intake will be an essential guide to treatment, equal in importance to the record of sugar in the urine," Dr. Joslin said. A week later the diet was reduced to 53 carbohydrate, 40 protein, and 17 fat, and that is only 525 calories, or about a third of what a man requires for his maintenance if he stays quiet in bed. Before insulin, the treatment of diabetes was far from satisfactory.

By October 27, two weeks later, the urine sugar was less and the blood sugar was down to 190 milligrams per 100 cubic centimeters. The diabetes was better, but the patient was miserable — literally starved — and he looked it. He had lost seven more pounds. On November 21, the diet was increased, and his weight rose again to 134, owing in part to the retention of extra fluid in the body. A good sign was that the blood sugar remained low at 150. The method of treatment by starvation and "rest to the pancreas," which Dr. Frederick M. Allen[2] and others had advocated, was heroic, but evidently it could pay off.

In February 1922, the diet contained nearly 2000 calories, but George's weight had fallen to 122 because of the loss of body water. The blood sugar still ranged around 150 milligrams per 100 cubic centimeters.

The diabetes was severe. Both George and Marian had courage — a much deeper courage than might have appeared from their reactions to getting wet in the rain or being disturbed by a draft of cold air. Marian's devoted service, amplified by her wisdom, her common sense, and her cheerful disposition, began early, and it continued. The fact that George kept going in spite of his handicap was due in large part to his remarkable wife.

Dorothy and I were seeing George and Marian at least every other week, and very little was ever said about diabetes. George never discussed the level of his blood sugar or his daily progress. We could see, of course, that he was in trouble; the loss of weight was obvious, but his spirits were good in spite of everything. There were times when he was short-tempered, but anyone who is half-starved and always hungry has a right to blow off steam now and then. George did "cheat" in one way: he learned later that alcohol was burned directly and not by conversion to sugar, and so he allowed himself a very dry Martini whenever there was an "occasion," like dining with friends.

When George and Marian traveled anywhere — even up the street to dine out — they brought along a little old black leather slouch bag, which had seen better days but was still all in one piece, It contained a Chatillon scales and a tin pie-plate, and, some time later, it contained the bottle of insulin, with the syringes, the alcohol, and the gauze sponges, not to mention the little block of blue paper and a couple of pencils. In helping himself to food, George put it first on the pie-plate, to adjust its weight on the scales before adding it to his dinner plate. The amount was noted on the blue paper, which he placed to one side. Often he would turn to Marian: "How much spinach, did you say? I have allowed for the cracker and the bit of cheese that I ate with the cocktail! I figured the cracker as five grams and the cheese at two grams — that's right, isn't it?" Marian could remember the values of food better than George could, and she knew what he should have. She was the one who tallied the blue papers at the end of the day and entered the total on the record.

For the rest of his life, George ate no food at all that was not weighed or measured and recorded. Later on, when he and Marian went to formal dinners, they did learn to estimate the quantities with some success. Marian's idea of asking the hostess ahead of time what the menu was going to be was often very helpful. If the hostess was surprised by the telephone call, she soon saw that with the advance information George could plan his intake more successfully.

Under ordinary circumstances, when at home and when dining with close friends, the scales, the tin pie-plate, and the little blue block were produced from the little old bag.

Meantime, a wonderful change was coming — insulin!

The discovery of insulin was very much a high point in medical progress. It was one of the first dramatic results of the new system of medical education that had been stimulated by the Flexner Report of 1910, twelve years before.

The reader must know that the pancreas — the sweetbread of the butcher shop — is the seat of trouble in diabetes. This essential organ has two kinds of cells, corresponding to its two main functions. The "external" secretion is poured into the intestine and helps to digest our food. The "internal" secretion, which is even more important, comes from special cells that can be seen in groups and are called the "islands of Langerhans." The secretion from these cells enters the blood stream directly, and is essential to the utilization of sugar by the body. When the pancreas is removed, "total diabetes" occurs at once, as von Mering and Minkowski first showed in 1889.

When a fresh, normal beef or hog pancreas is put through a meat grinder, and the pulp is mixed with water or with physiologic salt solution, or even with diluted alcohol, and is then filtered, the extract is toxic, because it contains split products of protein. Injections of it will reduce the blood sugar of a depancreatized animal, to be sure, but at the same time they will make the animal sick.

In May 1922, Dr. Frederick G. Banting, later Sir Frederick, made the dramatic report[3] to the meeting of the Association of American Physicians that he and his group of workers in Toronto had been able to obtain the internal secretion of the pancreas fairly free of the toxic material. In his discussion of Dr. Banting's paper, Dr. Frederick M. Allen, whose own studies on diabetes had been so extensive, hailed the result as "one of the greatest achievements of modern medicine."

How it had come about is an interesting story. In 1920, Dr. Banting had chanced to read a paper by Moses Barron,[4] in which Barron showed that the degenerative changes that follow blockage of the pancreatic duct by gallstones are quite the same as the changes that follow experimental ligation of the pancreatic duct. The assumption was that ligation would cause a greater degeneration of the islands of Langerhans than of the other (acinic) cells and that an extract of the degenerated pancreas would contain mostly the internal secretion.

Dr. Banting went to the University of Toronto to consult Professor J. J. R. MacLeod, and, after some delay, experiments were begun in May 1921. The placing of ligatures around the pancreatic duct of the laboratory dogs was difficult, but it was accomplished with the help of Mr. Charles H. Best, then a medical student. After some weeks, an extract of the pancreas from a "duct-tied" dog was obtained. This extract was still somewhat toxic, but it did reduce the blood sugar and save the life of a depancreatized animal. Dr. Joseph H. Pratt of Boston, himself a great student of diabetes, has said:

> It is fortunate that neither Dr. Moses Barron nor Dr. Banting realized that previous workers had shown that simple ligation [of the pancreatic duct] is not permanent because the proensymes in the pancreatic juice become activated by the injured tissue around the ligature and soon burrow a new passage into the intestine . . . Moreover, the temporary atrophy which everyone, including Banting, had observed, involves the acinic as well as the islet cells, and therefore the two parts of the pancreas are not separated by the procedure . . . Finally, the tabulation of Dr. Banting's own experiments shows all too clearly that extractions of the *normal* pancreas gave results which were quite as good as other extractions of his duct-tied "degenerated" pancreas.[5]

Dr. Banting and Mr. Best used alcohol for their extractions, even though Dr. Banting was wrong in his idea that alcohol would "suppress the toxic product." In the middle of their work Dr. James B. Collip, biological chemist, joined the team of Banting, Best, and MacLeod and in a very short time Dr. Collip made a critical observation.

When the mash of normal pancreas is treated with only half its volume of 95-percent alcohol, it is obvious that the mixture contains only about 30 percent of alcohol. One day, Dr. Collip filtered a quantity of this mixture and then poured the clear filtrate into four volumes of strong 95-percent alcohol. When he did this, a precipitate formed, and after he had collected it on a filter paper, he found that it was soluble in water. Then came the exciting experiment in which the team of workers found that the alcoholic precipitate, now redissolved in water, was extremely active in reducing the blood sugar of diabetic dogs. Equally important, it was not toxic. Dr. Collip had shown that in strong alcohol the toxic portion remains in solution while the active portion precipitates. Insulin had been isolated. (Since then, other investigators have shown that the important circumstance is not the alcohol so much as the isoelectric point. The process has been greatly simplified.)

On January 11, 1922, the first diabetic patients were treated with the new extract at the Toronto General Hospital. By February 22, 1922, the effects had been observed in seven patients, all of whom had done well. The sugar in both blood and urine was lowered, but the extracts contained so much protein that abscesses developed; the extracts were still too toxic. At that point, Professor MacLeod turned most of his staff over to the problem of purification, naming the new extract "insulin."

Through the spring the work continued, but the supply of insulin was limited, because Banting and Best had to make it themselves. In April 1922, however, the Eli Lilly Company, under the direction of Dr. G. H. A. Clowes, lent their resources to the problem, and plans for large-scale production were considered. It was not until August, however, that Banting and Best had a stock sufficient to send a small sample to Dr. Joslin in Boston. On August 7, 1922, Dr. Joslin first gave insulin to one of his patients, but some months passed before he had enough to give George Minot his first dose.

George was awfully thin. He was drinking black coffee in quantity and smoking many cigarettes in the effort to curb his appetite. He struggled to the hospital each day, but he was tired and irritable. He was allowed to eat only 1675 calories each day, and that was not enough to maintain proper nutrition. His weight was down to 120 pounds, and his blood sugar was up to 240 milligrams percent.

Finally the great day came. Dr. Joslin had at last been able to secure a little insulin for George, and on January 12, 1923, three doses, containing respectively 1, 2, and 3 units, were injected under the skin at intervals of six hours. By April, George's daily doses had gone up to 14 units, and at about that time the production of insulin on a commercial scale had been started by the Lilly Company. There was still sugar in George's urine, but he had gained five pounds, and he felt much better. All the rest of us felt better, too.

There is no doubt that this new treatment saved George Minot's life. Dr. Joslin's figures[6] showed clearly that diabetes coming on with that severity at that age would have been fatal in a relatively few years. After the start of treatment with insulin, George's physical condition improved almost at once, and, more important, his confidence in his own future welfare was restored. With insulin, he could see that his diabetes could be controlled, even if the business of measuring, recording, and regulating his food intake must be continued indefinitely. The discovery of insulin was directly responsible for George's being able to carry on and to make his own discovery of the treatment for pernicious anemia.

During 1923 and 1924, George was taking 18 units of insulin before breakfast and 12 units before dinner at night. Marian's note in May 1924, reads, "This is the first winter since marriage that he has not lost 7 to 21 days' work from illness."

Insulin reactions, due to the sudden burning of the sugar in the blood, lowering the concentrations beyond the safe limit, were not infrequent. They came more often when George was tired or when he had been exercising. The symptoms were evidently very troublesome, for he would exclaim, "Marian, please get me an orange or a couple of crackers, and get it quick! I am having a reaction!" George would appropriate the individual lumps of sugar wrapped in paper whenever he saw them in a hotel or a dining car. One or two of them were in his pocket at all times, but orange juice had a faster action.

Few people in those early days knew that George had diabetes. Francis Peabody knew, Reginald Fitz knew, and a few other close friends knew, but otherwise the diagnosis was kept secret. People at the Huntington saw George losing weight and looking tired, but the change was not sudden, and they thought that perhaps he was working too hard. When George left the Hospital earlier in the afternoon than usual, it was quite understandable.

It was not until 1918 that George's private practice even began to be an important item. He was interested much more in research and teaching than in making money. Seeing a few private patients gave him a chance to apply his knowledge, to broaden his experience, and to help the patient and the family doctor.

It was Dr. Edwin A. Locke who wanted George to do more in private practice. Dr. Locke was a tall, well-built, nicely dressed man who had developed a large practice among well-to-do people. Cousin Jim had watched him during Locke's house-pupil days at the Massachusetts General Hospital in 1902, and had recognized his good background and his pleasing personality. When Locke showed an interest in tuberculosis, Cousin Jim had him appointed to an assistantship at the Boston Consumptives' Hospital in Mattapan; and when Cousin Bessie died of pneumonia in 1903, Dr. Locke had stayed in the house and helped Cousin Jim during that dreadful time. Nine years later, when we were in medical school, Dr. Locke was Visiting Physician to the Boston City Hospital, where he taught practical medicine to a group of admiring students. Quite obviously, Dr. Locke knew all about George Minot, and relations between them now became close and intimate.

In September 1921, almost coincident with George's new job at the Huntington and the onset of his diabetes, Dr. Locke invited George and Dr. Gerald Blake to join him in forming the "311 Beacon Street" Group. Dr. Locke had plenty of room for offices on the two lower floors of his house at 311, and the place was only a block away from 188 Marlborough Street. To set up a good laboratory, to have secretaries and typewriters in common, as well as complete sets of medical journals, would lead to greater efficiency and economy for all concerned. If one man were away at a meeting, or on vacation, his patients would be taken care of. The idea was very appealing. Blake, Locke, and Minot — the names arranged alphabetically, were the Associates, and Articles of Agreement, concerned chiefly with the finances, were drawn up by a lawyer and signed by all parties. Dr. Donald S. King joined the group as Assistant, and later came Dr. James Hitchcock, Dr. William P. Murphy, Dr. George P. Reynolds, Dr. Richard B. King, Dr. Richard P. Stetson, and Dr. Francis T. Hunter — but that was some time later.

The laboratory was an important feature, and Dr. Locke was fortunate in securing the services of Mrs. Ouida C. Montague, a graduate of Simmons College, to take charge of it. Mrs. Montague was not only a competent chemist, but also she was easy to work with, and tactful and kind with the patients. Under the guidance of

George Minot, she became expert in the technique of blood examinations. For many years she gave devoted service to the doctors at 311 and to the many people who came to them for advice and treatment. Miss Frances Preble has been chief secretary to the 311 group for twenty-five years, first with Dr. Locke, then with Dr. Minot, and now with Dr. Stetson.

Private patients received excellent care from George Minot. He spent a long time with the histories; every detail of the symptoms was noted. Always, he was curious to learn what sort of person the patient was; where he or she lived; what he or she did all day; whether life was happy and congenial or whether conditions in the family were difficult in some way. And then, above all, he would ask, "Tell me about your diet. What do you have for breakfast? Where do you eat breakfast? Must you catch a train shortly afterwards — and do you rush for it — or can you sit for a minute and then walk to the station comfortably and at ease?" The study of the total food intake was usually of paramount importance: "Do you eat meat every day? What kind of meat, and how much of it? What about milk and eggs and vegetables and fruit? And how are these latter prepared?" And, finally: "Do you enjoy your meals or do you eat because you feel that you have to eat?"

As has been said, George learned, in the very beginning, that deficiencies in the total diet were common, especially in the patients with anemias, and as time passed he came to think ever more and more about food. The questions about the mode of life were important also. The answers gave him an insight into the character of the individual and into problems that might complicate an otherwise simple picture.

I can recall two cases that pleased George, because it was his meticulous history — his recording of every little detail — that gave him the clue to the diagnoses. The first case was that of a rather stout, middle-aged Jewish woman who had been coming to the Out-Patient Department at the M.G.H. for years. Her hospital record was at least two inches thick. She had been seen in every clinic, for she had symptoms in every part of her body. George found three things wrong with her. The first was that her home life was dreadful. The husband was sick and unable to work, and neither she nor he knew how to cope with his troubles. The oldest child was married and too busy with her family to pay attention to the old folks; the other three children were in their teens and quite out of the mother's control. Second, her diet was poor. She lived mostly on sugars and starches, taking very little meat — "chicken soup sometimes" — very few vegetables, and no fruit. Moreover, the meals were irregular, eaten at odd times, "when I get hungry," and eaten mostly by herself. The setting was far from congenial. It was not surprising, therefore, that, thirdly, she had anemia — the hemoglobin down to 60 percent and the red count low at 3.5 million. To persuade the husband to come in for examination was hard, but finally he arrived, and was found to have tuberculosis. He was sent to a sanitarium, where he did very well, and that relieved a heavy burden at home. To persuade the patient to eat a decent diet and to change her habits of eating so as to enjoy her food and her children at the same time was also hard. The directions had to be repeated many times. Fortunately, however, George Minot gained her confidence. Slowly but surely she learned the lesson; she lost some of her fat and gained color. Her sense of well-being improved greatly and most of her symptoms disappeared. She stopped going to the other clinics.

The second patient was a private one. She had been seen by "all the doctors" in Baltimore, Philadelphia, and New York, some of them well known, but she came to Boston to have Doctor Minot treat her anemia. The history was long and complicated; "indigestion" and "weakness" were the chief symptoms. Gross examination showed nothing very wrong, except a moderate anemia of the secondary type. George asked more about the indigestion — all the details about pains and gas, as well as about her food and eating habits. In 1921 x-rays were not taken with the ease and freedom that are enjoyed today, but, nevertheless, this lady had had an x-ray examination of her stomach, without any abnormalities being found. As George studied her history, he became convinced that gallstones, with an infection in the gall bladder, might be causing her anemia, and so her symptoms. A new x-ray showed trouble in the gall bladder; at operation a dozen stones were found and removed, and the lady was cured. The aftermath was amusing — or was it pathetic? Her surgeon sent a bill for $1000 and received his check promptly. George Minot sent a bill for $100 and received an indignant letter: "You did not cure me; it was Dr. X who removed my disease." George told me later that it took not a little persuasion to make the lady understand that, of all the doctors whom she had seen in times past, only he had been thorough enough to take a really complete history, which, by itself, revealed the nature of her difficulty. He got his money, and the lady got a little understanding of the importance of a thorough, competent study if a good diagnosis is to be made. She learned more later, for some years afterward she made a handsome contribution toward the support of his laboratory, and that was something that George appreciated immensely.

To say that George was a good doctor is trite enough. His love for people, especially his patients, was unusual. He took good care *of* his patients because he cared *for* his patients, as Francis Peabody expressed it. More than one friend has stopped me to inquire about him. For example one asked: "How is Dr. Minot? He looks tired. If he worries about other people the way he worried about my John and about me, he should be tired. You can have no idea of his utter devotion to us. We all knew that leukemia was a fatal disease, but he was so cheerful and encouraging about it, and at the same time so sincere and so honest, that John would brighten up whenever Dr. Minot came to the house. And as for me, I do not know how I could have stood the strain without the moral support which he gave me. He was indeed a real friend."

When this particular "John" died, George was quite disturbed by the failure of all the new drugs, and of all the latest forms of treatment, to help the man. The demand to learn more about leukemia became even more insistent.

In 1921 and 1922 George published papers as usual, most of them clinical papers, describing cases that illustrated the different forms of leukemia and anemia. Dr. Henry A. Christian had undertaken to revise the old *Oxford Medicine* in several volumes, and he asked George to write the "Clinical Discussion of the Anemias." [7] It took both time and energy to write the necessary ninety pages. In 1920, Thomas Nelson and Sons of New York had brought out a new form of textbook. *The Nelson Loose-Leaf Living Medicine* had pages that could be removed and replaced from time to time as new knowledge might develop. This idea appealed to George, and he worked with Dr. Roger I. Lee on the chapters concerned with the blood and its diseases.[8] Meantime, a compendium on *Endocrinology and Metabolism,* edited by Dr. Lewellys F. Barker of Baltimore, appeared, with George and Dr. Arlie V. Bock writing the section on transfusion.[9]

Success in medicine carries a penalty; or one should say that the opportunity for investigation, and the brilliance of mind that makes investigation fruitful, carry the obligation to share the new knowledge with others. As George grew in scientific stature, he was beset with more and more invitations to speak before medical societies, small and large, local and national, and, more troublesome, he had to write dissertations and review articles. Although these obligations are penalties insofar as they require time and energy needed badly for more investigation, it is only fair to note that they are part of the teaching function.

That George did find time goes without saying — and he needed a good deal of time if one is to judge from the notes that are still in his file. His talks were never casual; each one had to be prepared with care. "No, I am sorry that we cannot dine with you tomorrow, for George has a lecture on the day after, and his evening must be quiet and peaceful," Marian would explain. As a result of her care of him and his care of his preparation, George's talks were good.

The teaching of students was to George Minot a function of primary importance. Most of his informal lectures included references to simple principles. He often recalled the time when a House Pupil asked Dr. Frederick C. Shattuck to see "an ulcer."

"Young man," Dr. Shattuck turned on him, "if you are thinking about a patient, don't you ever call him an ulcer again."

"No, gentlemen," George would go on, after quoting Dr. Shattuck, "the patient is a whole person. What sort of person is he? Where does he live? Whom does he live with and what sort of place is his home? What does he do? Is his life easy or hard, and how does he take it? These are the things that we want to know!"

George was clear about physical examinations: "The modern tendency is to forget the value of the simplest procedures. Auscultation and not the x-ray is the first step in examining a chest," and "Studying his blood does not study the patient."

He warned against the pitfalls of drawing hasty conclusions

about the results of treatment. In one lecture he said, "To determine the true benefits of therapy is one of the most difficult tasks of modern medicine. [The difficulty] . . . depends on the variations in . . . the disease and it depends on the variations in . . . the patient; in his susceptibility — whether to disease or remedy."

"Never neglect the control," he said; "that important control 'Health' — a study of which is playing a large role in the progress of medicine today."

He was pleased when the small voice in the back row asked, "What would have happened to the patient if the doctor had not given him any drugs at all?"

"That," said George, "was one of the best and most pertinent discussions ever contributed!"

His ideas on teaching were sound. He believed that each student should be assigned a special topic on which to work, and that he should present his results in the form of a short paper to be delivered before a group of colleagues without reference to his notes. George thought that the topics should deal with principles rather than with diseases; with the functions of the stomach and their alterations rather than with gastric disease, or with jaundice rather than with liver disease. He used to say that, "The ways of approach to the patient and the value of common sense often are not adequately taught. Too many recent graduates have little idea how to take care of patients except in the wards of a hospital. They blunder in handling people." [10]

In October 1923, George and Marian moved their family from 247 Beacon Street to 30 Marlborough Street, which they bought and where they lived for six years.

George's teaching and research were going on together, as always. In 1923, Dr. Raphael Isaacs came to the Huntington to work full time on the biology of the blood cells. One problem concerned the mechanism by which the red cells matured in the bone marrow. Another concerned the behavior of the cells in a tumor called lymphoblastoma. Dr. Duane's high-voltage x-ray machine used in the treatment of tumors was producing mild radiation burns. It was important to study the mode of this action, but it was more important to learn the precautions necessary to prevent injury to both patient and doctor. This was done.

On December 6, 1923, the Huntington Medical Service was invited to present papers before the New York Academy of Medicine. Dr. William B. Castle, who worked with George for many years, has said that the reports of Minot, Buckman, and Isaacs on chronic myelogenous leukemia,[11] lymphatic leukemia,[12] and lymphoblastoma[13] are still standard references.

A good part of the financial support of George's laboratory came from the Medical School, which had made him a grant from the Proctor Fund. Dr. Joslin's aunt, Miss Ellen Proctor, had become interested in the possibilities of medical research through helping her nephew, then a medical student, translate from the German the classic paper on diabetes by von Mering and Minkowski.[14] She bequeathed $50,000 to the Medical School, and President Eliot of Harvard suggested the broad definition of its purposes: "For the Study of Chronic Diseases." A few years later, one of her nephews, Mr. Abel H. Proctor, added another $50,000. When, later on, George Minot's work involved the study of patients in several different hospitals, the wisdom of the broad objects of the Proctor Fund was appreciated. The last substantial grant terminated in October 1924, and George was worried. Where would he get the money for his assistants and the technicians? At that moment the situation was really serious, for it looked as if some of the work might have to be curtailed. George was concerned. He talked about contributing a thousand dollars from his own salary, and later he did give $1,500. He wrote to Dr. Locke: "If I can get a gift back, it will help. I have no idea how I can afford to give up to $1,500 but we are cancelling our plans for vacation on the Cape this summer and will live in Milton with my father so as to make the Huntington go."

The big trouble was that the Harvard Medical School could not contribute its own unrestricted funds, because the Huntington was under the Cancer Commission's control rather than under the Medical School, and the Cancer Commission itself did not have any extra money. Somehow or other, however, the difficulties were overcome, presumably through the wizardries of Dr. Edsall, who was now Dean of the Medical School. Perhaps the "gift" came in, for in the summer of 1925, George and Marian rented a house at Northeast Harbor, Maine, and invited Dorothy and me to spend a week with them there. All was well after all!

George was always thoughtful about his assistants. He selected them with care, and he wanted them to do well. How many employers will take the trouble to write to a new employee as George wrote in 1926 to this Simmons College graduate who was to come to work for him as a technician:

Dear Miss E——,

It is a pleasure to know that you will begin work October 11 . . . First of all, bear in mind that I wish everyone associated with the Medical Service of the Huntington Hospital to feel that he or she is a real part of the service and not purely an employee. As time passes by, and as you learn more and more, we may anticipate that you will be given increasing responsibilities and eventually consider taking up some actual investigative work. Please realize that there will be lots that can be done, and our spirit is to do all that we can, and do it well. Although your official hours are to be 9 to 5 . . . I want you to feel that should certain circumstances arise which might make you wish to arrive late or leave early, you may do so. I simply ask that such liberties are not taken constantly. Occasionally the work may be unduly pressing, and you might be expected to remain until 5:30 P.M. On other days, when the work is light, you might leave before 5 P.M.

He wrote to a doctor. After beginning, "Dear Dr. J——: It is a great pleasure to me to have you accept the appointment at the 'Huntington,'" he went on for four pages to tell the man about his duties and to make suggestions about the work.

Dr. Minot's section of the Hospital's Thirteenth Report (July 1, 1925) begins:

The modern laboratory does not supply something absolute which does away with the necessity for careful clinical study. Work emerging from it aids our understanding of disease. However, the care of the sick is the fundamental function of any hospital, and the teaching of medicine and research are important additional functions of a university hospital. Such is the nature of the work of the medical service and its laboratories.

Fifteen papers from the medical service were published in 1925. The Report goes on:

The teaching of medical students by Drs. Minot and Isaacs has been [continued] . . . with the addition of a volunteer course in June and a course for Naval graduate students during the spring . . . [Dr. Minot is pleased to announce that] Dr. Cyrus C. Sturgis [will be] Assistant Physician for the ensuing year . . . Dr. Minot has continued to give not less than one-half his time to work pertaining to the hospital. The time taken for supervision of the work indicated above, formulation of problems, editorial revision of manuscripts, etc., is considerable. Dr. Christian has most kindly made it possible for liaison with the Peter Bent Brigham Hospital, and Dr. Minot has been appointed Associate in Medicine at that institution.

George had much too many things to think about, and many of them were causes of real anxiety. Dr. Beth Vincent wanted him to write a paper on chronic thrombopenic purpura for the Congress of American Physicians and Surgeons. George wrote to Dr. Locke: "To do the paper the way I should like is a long job: the way he [Vincent] has in mind is casual. It will take me about 60 hours, I imagine, to do it properly. Do you advise that I make the time for it? Or shall I let it go?" He had seen only one private patient that week and was troubled by the lack of income, as well as by the difficulties at the Huntington. "I am tired, cross and upset," he wrote to Locke. "All my irons are in the fire, and none of them gets hot."

He had accepted invitations to speak in Hartford, Rochester, and Fall River. He needed intelligent help, a secretary who could look up references in the library. Dr. Locke's secretary could have done it, but she was too busy, and George did not like that. He found fault with the service at 311, but Locke reminded him that he was already using more of the laboratories and more secretarial help than any of the other associates, including Locke himself.

There was one pleasant event; George's brother Henry was married to Miss Ellen Sears Curtis on Saturday, October 18, 1924. The two families were at the reception in goodly numbers; two of Cousin Jim's sisters had died, but Aunt Louisa, eighty-three, Aunt Hattie, eighty-one, and Aunt Bessie, seventy-three, were well able to enjoy the festivities. The Minot family was a closely knit organization, each member proud of his or her association with the others. The Sunday night suppers, where the whole family met, either at 188, or at the Aunts', or at each others' houses, continued, with the children joining the group when they became old enough. These gatherings continued with fair regularity until 1942, when the Jimmy Minot family moved out of Boston to live permanently in Beverly.

The winter of 1924–25 was hard for George. He was always tired, but when he dined with us, or we with him, he would be cheerful and full of talk, as always. This talk was apt to be more about men than about strictly medical problems, but occasionally George would allude to pernicious anemia. "It looks as though the trouble had a good deal to do with the maturation of red cells. Why is it, do you suppose, that at certain times the bone marrow lies down on the job? We must find some way to study the function of the bone marrow. You know, I am always thinking about diet. It is food that makes different people different, and I have a good notion that the bone marrow needs food of some special sort."

In July 1925, when George was visiting every other day on the wards at the Peter Bent Brigham, working at the Huntington, and then seeing patients in his office, he was fairly well in spite of the heavy schedule. His weight was up to 140, the urine sometimes free of sugar, sometimes containing 1 percent. His blood sugar, however, was always high, sometimes over 300 milligrams per 100 cubic centimeters. Various experiments with both diet and insulin were made — a small extra dose of insulin was tried at bedtime, and then in March 1926, four daily doses in place of two were prescribed.,

His feet and legs bothered him from the beginning. Even before the onset of diabetes, George had complained of cold feet, particularly the left foot, which would develop a numbness and then begin to ache, evidently with some severity. The pain could be relieved by heat, and quite often he would take off his shoe and would hold his foot in front of his electric sun bowl or in front of the open fire. He had been warned about the risk of burning his numb toe. Other diabetic patients had had similar aches in their feet, and when they burned their toes, the complication was not only troublesome but dangerous, because gangrene had developed in one or two of these cases.

George's "indigestion" was still troublesome. He had pain, which evidently came in spasms, sometimes bad enough to make him press on his abdomen with his arms folded. There was no nausea and never any vomiting, and the pain was not related to meals. His own theory was that it was concerned with the pancreas, but there was no good evidence to support the idea. In November 1928, Dr. Chester M. Jones found that George's stomach contained less than the normal amount of acid, but what that had to do with the pain was not clear.

On the whole, however, George was all right. Certainly he was able to carry a heavy schedule, and carry it well, even though each night he was exhausted. And he was beginning to realize that his observations on the effect of diet in pernicious anemia were lending strong support to his theories, and that an announcement of results might be made fairly soon.

8

Pernicious Anemia

Bill Homans, George's classmate and fellow member of the "Edgartown High School," met George one day as he was walking down Marlborough Street. It was in December 1925, and it was cold and raw. George was bundled up in the long double-breasted black ulster coat that he wore on bad days. The coat went down to his ankles below, and up to the brim of his hat above. The old felt hat — it was the only hat he owned — was pulled down over his forehead, and the woolen muffler around his neck covered his chin as well. Tall and bent, with his head down and his hands in his pockets, he looked quite the opposite of dapper. Homans stopped him. "Hello," he said, "you look as though you were thinking about something quite hard — look out that you don't get run over when you cross the street. How are you anyway, and what's new?"

"Well, I'll tell you," George said. "You're right, I am thinking about something, and you are quite right about crossing the street. Back there I was too busy to look and a delivery truck almost hit me. Yes! I do have an idea — and I wish I could tell you about it!"

"Is your idea any good?" Homans asked.

"Well," he said, "maybe it's worth a nickel; maybe it's worth more than that!"

One night at about that time, when we were sitting after dinner at our house, George talked to me. "You know," he said, "that pernicious anemia is a disease which is fatal invariably. Patients who develop it live for only a few years. I keep thinking that the diet may have something to do with the cause. As I look at the smears of the blood in my patients, the microscope shows that in P.A. the red cells are not uniform as in the normal; they vary a good deal in their sizes and shapes and in their ability to take up stain. Occasionally one sees a cell with the nucleus intact, and that's a normoblast, of course, or one sees only a small dark spot — and that's a Howell-Jolly body. My idea is that these variations represent different stages in the development of the red cells, and they indicate that something is the matter with the bone marrow; it is not working properly, and the disease pernicious anemia depends upon a disturbance of bone-marrow function, which results in blood cells inferior both in quality and in quantity."

"Well! What causes that?" I broke in.

"Quite right," he said. "That's the question. I believe that the bone marrow needs food of some special kind. In other words, our patients with P.A. are deficient in some item in their total food intake.

"Do you remember meeting Dr. George H. Whipple of Rochester at Atlantic City? He is a big man, very pleasant, and easy to talk with. Whipple tells me — and his papers report it — that in his dogs made anemic by repeated bleedings, recovery of the blood count and of the hemoglobin blood color is more rapid if the dogs are given a diet which contains liver among other ingredients, and I will tell you about that in a minute.

"First, though, I must say how lucky we are to have Bill Murphy. He is a terrific worker, and I have got him counting reticulocytes on a number of our patients in the [Peter Bent] Brigham Hospital. We are finding that the 'retics' give us a good measure of bone-marrow function. When their numbers in the blood smear go up, we know that the bone marrow is being stimulated, and so, you see, we have a method by which the effect of treatment — any treatment — can be investigated.

"Now then, acting on the suggestion in Whipple's work, we have been giving liver to our patients, and some of them are really better. And we know they are better, because their reticulocytes shoot up within four or five days after the liver diet is started, and then of course the total red count and the hemoglobin follow soon after."

"How much liver do you give them?" I asked.

"Ah!" he said with a little smile of satitsfaction, "the patient who did best was a man who really liked liver. When he asked if he could take all the liver he wanted, I said 'Sure, of course' — and you should have seen him eat liver! And goodness me, the 'retic' response in his case was extraordinary. Now we are trying hard to follow up what this case taught us. We try to persuade every patient to eat liver up to at least a half pound a day — and more if possible. It's a lot of liver, but they eat it."

Dr. William B. Castle has written a good paragraph about the secret of George's success:

> That his own capacity for taking infinite pains was the right prescription for his genius is clear from the fact that, although the idea of a relation between good food and good blood was "in the air" and had been brought down to earth by the fundamental work of Whipple and his associates, many physicians fed diets containing liver to patients with pernicious anemia without being convinced, or at least without convincing others, of their value. Only Minot had the instincts and the persistence essential for clear-cut success. Thus, he was prepared to believe that the characteristic remissions of the disease were not "spontaneous." He detected the first slight clinical signs of improvement that followed a change in diet . . . Together with Dr. W. P. Murphy, he increased the amount of liver to an "optimal" though sometimes nauseating daily amount, and demonstrated over and over again the sequence of liver feeding, beginning clinical improvement, reticulocyte response and subsequent progressive rise of red-cell and hemoglobin levels. . . .
>
> Looking back, one finds it difficult to understand why this great clinical discovery, made in the end by such simple means, was delayed until well into the twentieth century. Probably, this was because, at last, in their own consistently successful dietary regimen, Minot and Murphy knowingly took no chances of inadequacy of dosage or of omitting possible essentials. Apparently in order of importance in their minds was the daily ingestion of 100 to 240 gm. of liver, 120 gm. of "muscle meat," leafy vegetables, especially lettuce and spinach, fruit, eggs, and milk. The diet was designed to be "rich in iron and purine derivatives." Fortunately, liver, which must have been chiefly advantageous in the hypochromic anemias of Whipple's dogs because of its iron content, was, as is now realized, also a good source of vitamin B_{12} and of folic acid. All but 3 of the first 45 patients also received hydrochloric acid, but it was noted that these 3 "improved at least as much as the majority of the others." After admitting that the consistent remissions in their own series of cases "may not last longer than those of others," they conservatively "urged pernicious anemia patients to take a diet of the sort described." [1]

All through the winter and spring, Minot and Murphy worked hard. The treatment of their patients was uniformly successful. In each case the liver diet produced a rise in reticulocytes, and that was followed by great clinical improvement.

George had been talking with Reginald Fitz, his great friend who was a physician at the Brigham, concerning a presentation of the results to the Association of American Physicians at their meeting in Atlantic City in May. If Minot and Murphy would describe the clinical aspects, then Fitz, Murphy, and Monroe could talk about the physiological side of the matter — to explain the function of the bone marrow, the maturation of the various cells, and then the effect of liver on these functions. They could report on a total of 45 cases, all with good "work-ups." The blood, as well as the general clinical conditions of the patients, had been followed closely and, as George said, "it ought not to be too difficult to put them all together."

On Tuesday, May 4, 1926, at the Traymore Hotel in Atlantic City, the last paper on the morning program of the Association meeting was entitled "Observations on Patients with Pernicious Anemia Partaking of a Special Diet." This paper was divided into two parts — "A. Clinical Aspects" by George R. Minot, M.D., and William P. Murphy, M.D. (By Invitation),* which was read by George; and "B. Physiological Aspects" by William P. Murphy, M.D. (By Invitation), Reginald Fitz, M.D., and Robert D. Monroe, M.D. (By Invitation), which was read by Fitz. Minot and Murphy reported their results on the forty-five cases. Listen to these quotations, taken from the complete paper published soon after the meeting.

> While the problem of diet in the treatment of pernicious anemia is by no means new, in our opinion its possible importance has not heretofore been generally recognized.

> In spite of attention to diet for the anemic patient, the influence of food on blood formation and destruction has received comparatively little consideration, and special sorts of food, because of some particular effect, have seldom been chosen for patients with pernicious anemia.

> The condition of all forty-five patients became much better rather rapidly soon after commencing the diet. All except one, who has recently omitted her diet, are now at the least in a very fair state of health, and if it were not for disorders in some due to spinal cord lesions, would

* "By Invitation" means that the coauthor of the paper was not a member of the Association.

have an appearance to a layman of being essentially well. However, there are only eleven patients who began the diet a year or more ago, two of whom have taken it for more than two years. Eighteen began taking the diet less than five months ago.

Clinical improvement has been obvious usually within two weeks. This has been heralded in the peripheral blood before the end of the first week by the beginning of a most definite rise of the reticulocytes . . . of from about 1.0 percent to usually about 8.0 and even to 15.5 percent of all the red blood cells.

The spontaneous remissions of pernicious anemia and the bizarre course it often runs make it notoriously difficult to determine accurately the effect of any procedure on the disease. All sorts of therapeutic procedures have been advised, many because a few cases improved promptly after their trial. Waves of enthusiasm for certain methods have vanished soon when it was shown that the earlier reports of benefit could be attributed readily to the natural course of the disease. There is, however, no doubt, as shown by some of the early and more recent investigators, that a well-balanced, nutritious diet sometimes aids to enhance a remission. The patient may be helped by numerous other forms of treatment, such as those to change the intestinal flora, the injection of protein substances, the taking of arsenic, the transfusion of blood, and splenectomy.

The evidence at hand suggests that the dietetic treatment of pernicious anemia is of considerable importance. It has been possible to demonstrate in forty-five cases, seen essentially in sequence, that following a diet rich in liver and low in fat a distinct remission of the anemia occurs rather promptly. The promptness and rapidity with which the red blood corpuscles and hemoglobin increased, coincident with at least rather marked subjective improvement in the sense of well-being and clinical appearance of all the patients and the strikingly better health of many, is at least unusual in pernicious anemia. It is also not customary for the red blood cell counts during remissions of pernicious anemia to be so frequently of the height that occurred in these patients. We are inclined to believe that something contained in the foods rich in complete proteins is particularly responsible for the improvement of the state of the blood.

It is possible that this series of cases eventually may be proved to be unusual in that there happened to be treated a group that would have taken a turn for the better under other circumstances. Also, time may show that the special diet used, of liver and similar food, is no more advantageous in the treatment of pernicious anemia than any ordinary nutritious diet. Let this be as it may, at the present time it seems to us, as it has to Gibson and Howard, that it is wise to urge pernicious anemia patients to take a diet of the sort described.[2]

How cautious George was about making any claim that he could not support!

I remember that meeting well. I can still see George, tall and very thin, on the platform in the Traymore Hotel, standing very erect behind the lectern, his face tense and his eyes wide open. He was talking very earnestly, choosing his words with greatest care; he had to share his time limit of fifteen minutes with Fitz. Behind him was the President, Dr. Richard P. Strong, and the Secretary, Dr. Francis W. Peabody, sitting back of the green beige table. In front were about five hundred physicians, many of them distinguished professors of medicine, assembled from all parts of the United States and Canada. Younger men were there, too, for the meetings are open to all.

I can still hear the applause, and I can see George stepping down off the platform with a smile on his face, obviously flattered by the generous reception and relieved that the job had been done and had evidently been done well. It was an exciting moment, and when the morning session ended, everyone wanted to extend his congratulations to George. Marian, squeezed into the back row, was pleased, too. That night, at the Association Dinner, George sat at Dr. Strong's head table. He was in great form, laughing and joking with everybody.

The news spread fast. Dr. Locke was at the meeting, but even so he sent a note afterwards to George:

"We are all thrilled by the results of the P.A. paper, and I join in the congratulations. Very pleasant things are being said, especially about your moderate claims. I thought you had as good if not better a handout as did any other report. Such work as Murphy has been doing this winter is what counts — the conscientious, thorough study of the cases. You must not let the tide swamp you."

It was hard to believe that this man, George Minot, who three years before had been in real danger of death from diabetes and whose life had been saved by one very recent medical discovery, should have had the courage and the fortitude, as well as the supreme intelligence, to collect and present the evidence for another major discovery which was destined to abolish another dreadful disease, pernicious anemia, as a cause of death.

On the morning after the meeting, Dr. Henry A. Marble, a surgical friend of ours, was working at the Chelsea Hospital on a poor old man, obviously in his last illness. He was getting ready to give the man one more of the transfusions that Dr. George Minot had advised. The old man was saying, "What is the use of all this fuss when I will be dead so soon?" Just then the door opened and a young doctor burst in: "Mr. X, did you see the morning paper? Dr. Minot has found the cure for pernicious anemia." Right then and there the old man was made to eat liver. Within a week he was much better, and eventually he recovered completely.

Dr. Francis T. Hunter has described, in Dr. Washburn's book, the first case of pernicious anemia ever cured at the Massachusetts General Hospital:

> When I was a Senior, in the spring of 1926, George Minot one Sunday at lunch whispered in my ear to try large amounts of liver on the next pernicious anemia case I had. I can recall the patient very clearly, as I have seen him in the past month [twenty-eight years after his first treatment] in the Out-Patient Department. He was a retired actor.
>
> He came in to the Hospital with a red count of less than 1,000,000, practically moribund and with a patch of bronchopneumonia. His wife gave him one transfusion, and there was $25 left in the family [sugar bowl] with which to bury him. Bill Salter was the "pup" at the time and was very disgusted at my ordering him to get a meat-grinder, grind up tons of liver every day, and to pump it into this man with a nasal tube. He did it, however, and for several days nothing happened. The patient seemed to be getting worse. I recall sitting on the steps of the Bulfinch Building about one o'clock one morning with Walter Bauer, arguing as to whether we would take the family's $25 for another transfusion or use it to bury the patient. We finally decided to give him one more transfusion. This was done and about 48 hours later . . . [the patient] came out of his coma rather suddenly and, swearing in a rather feeble voice, complained that this was "a hell of a place where they didn't give you enough to eat." He progressively and rapidly got better, and we were so proud of him that he was kept on the ward for the next three months.[3]

As his paper demonstrates, George Minot had been treating patients with liver for some time, a few for as long as two years before his report was released. It interests me to find that the notes of the Medical Exchange Club meeting, held at George's house on February 16, 1926, which was less than three months prior to the reading of his paper in Atlantic City, say almost nothing about this new treatment — and this is in spite of the fact that he was talking only to his intimate friends.

The last sentence of the Medical Exchange Club notes does, however, say this: "Other topics under active investigation at the Huntington Hospital include: Diagnosis by studying vitally stained material obtained by lymph node puncture; the sugar metabolism of tumors; the development of a microspirometer, and The Influence of Diet on Blood Production and Cell Growth." One has to wonder whether up to that time George himself realized the full significance of his finding, and Locke's expression about George's presentation in Atlantic City, "as good if not better a handout," does not signify an appreciation that was basic and fundamental.

There is another item. On April 28, 1926, only six days before the meeting in Atlantic City, George gave a talk on pernicious anemia at the Boston Medical Library, and he must have smiled to himself as he went along. The notes of this talk are in their own folder, and both the notes and the folder show the date; evidently he thought of it as an important communication. "The patient with P.A. is thought of as being sick. The color of the skin is comparable to the color of a grapefruit. The Clinical picture is one of weakness and debility . . . A constitutional type is often seen in that most of these patients have a large, bulky frame. Heredity may be important . . . The course of the disease is downhill . . . There is a lack of acid in the stomach . . . Lesions of the nervous system may develop later." Not one word was said about diet; nothing whatever about treatment, nothing about the forty-five cases, not even "the hope that studies now going on might bring interesting results." It is hard to know why he held back to this extent. Of course he wanted to make his real announcement before the Association of American Physicians, but he might have given the Suffolk District Medical Society just a little hint — at least a hope!

At the Exchange Club, on February 16, he did talk about the normal day-to-day variation in the blood counts, as demonstrated by Richard P. Stetson, at that time a fourth-year medical student, and he talked about the size of the red cells: that young cells are larger than old cells. Today one talks about the hematocrit — the relative volume of the red cells packed in the bottom of the tube after centrifugation under standard conditions — and one talks also about the mean corpuscular volume — a figure obtained by dividing the hematocrit times ten by the number of millions in the red-cell count.

A few days after their complete paper was published, in the *Journal of the American Medical Association,* Murphy and Minot wrote in the *Boston Medical and Surgical Journal* for August 26:

> In the issue [of the *J.A.M.A.*] of August 14, 1926 . . . we reported upon the distinct improvement in the health of patients with pernicious anemia, partaking of a special diet . . . In order that physicians may advise readily this diet for patients, it is described below in greater detail than in the paper referred to above . . . The daily requirements of the diet in order of assumed importance are:[4]

— and the list begins with liver (calves, beef, chicken) or kidneys (lamb) freshly cooked — at least 120 gm., preferably 200 gm. or more (cooked weight).

After the discovery of the effect of whole liver on the function of the bone marrow, and consequently on the clinical course of pernicious anemia, the next step was to try to purify the liver, partly to learn about the manner of its action, and particularly to simplify and perhaps standardize the use of liver in the treatment of patients. Dr. Edwin J. Cohn, Professor of Physical Chemistry at the Harvard Medical School, had the knowledge and the equipment, and above all the experience required to separate protein substances one from another, and George went to him. This is the same Dr. Cohn who some years later showed how to isolate gamma globulin from the blood. George's demonstration that the percentage of reticulocytes in the blood smear provided an index of bone-marrow activity implied that the "reticulocyte response" could be used as a guide for the clinical testing of whatever fraction Dr. Cohn might produce. To have such a test as this made the plan of attack easy to foresee: Dr. Cohn must make the fractions and then Dr. Minot must develop his organization so that the testing of each product could be well executed and well controlled, using each time a number of patients with pernicious anemia who would presumably give positive results, and other patients with anemia of other kinds who would presumably give negative results.

Almost at once Cohn showed that it was a simple matter to eliminate a great mass of liver protein and leave the active principle in a relatively small residue which came to be known as "Fraction G." When the news about this Fraction G. was heard by outside practitioners, George's telephone began to ring: "Please, oh please, can you let me have just enough of your wonderful product to treat my very sick patient?" For a moment it looked as though Harvard University, under Dr. Cohn, was about to engage in the pharmaceutical business, and when the calls became more numerous and more insistent, George, and Dr. Cohn too, became quite excited and worried about it. Here was something that George had not anticipated, and he went to Dr. Edsall and later to President Lowell to ask their help and advice. Mr. Lowell agreed that production must be controlled and supervised if material of inferior quality was not to find its way to patients. The upshot was that a committee was formed to study the matter, and in a few weeks a patent was applied for in the name of Harvard University. When the license to manufacture was granted, the condition was added that each lot should be tested clinically under the direction of the Committee. When one large lot was found to be quite inert, the wisdom of the condition was demonstrated.

These "legal affairs" sounded ominous, if not frightening, to George, but when he saw an advertisement which showed that "Liver Extract" was being offered for sale by a company that George had never heard of, he was very indignant. "It makes me hot," he said, and added, "Please see that the Committee considers whether any action should or could be taken." The episode convinced him that "legal affairs" were important after all.

In the meantime, through the interest and the courtesy of Dr. G. H. A. Clowes, Medical Director of the Eli Lilly Company, it was arranged that the Lilly Company should be given the exclusive rights to the manufacture of Cohn's "Fraction G.," or "Lilly 343" as they called it at first.

The testing of the fraction was easy in theory, but not so easy in practice. Dr. Herman A. Lawson was Resident Physician at the

Huntington for the year beginning October 1, 1926, at precisely the time when the testing was at its height. One day a large bottle full of a reddish, thick, soupy material was sent over from Cohn's laboratory. Lawson thought it was "an awful looking mess," but he found a "note" — four pages in longhand — from George:

Dear Lawson, The liver mess is in the icebox in the Huntington kitchen: it contains the liver proteins left over after the extraction of what we think is the active material, and we must prove that it has no value — no ability to produce a retic response. Please see that Mike C—— receives 250 Grams of the stuff each day, and I want you personally to see that he swallows it. Get Miss Connover to spice it up and butter it — put lemon in it — do anything she can think of to make it go, but go it must. Maybe a sprig of parsley on the side would help some. C—— must get it down somehow — and we will hope that he can keep it down. After he eats it, count the reticulocytes twice every day, and keep your records carefully. We do not expect a rise, but we might get one if Cohn's extraction has not been complete, or perhaps we will find that the do-good is present in some other part of the liver as well as in Fraction G.

Meantime, Mr. E. at the Phillips House [Private Ward of the Massachusetts General Hospital] is getting the bitter fraction of D, and A on Ward A. is getting the other half of D. The technician at the M.G.H. can do the lab work all right, but it is up to you to see that she does it, and also that she gets the red counts and the hemoglobin. Be sure that the [blood] smears are good: keep them on file and be sure they are labelled and dated. As for Mr. W. on Ward F, see that Murphy supplies you every other day with the exact amount of liver pulp undiluted and get Murphy to collect the smears for the retics daily.

And then George adds: "This sounds 'military' but it is not. You are doing excellently and are mixed up with *Big Things* — Good!"

Another message said:

Tell Lawson that the chances of a lifetime are at hand. An excellent new patient is on the way. His name is Mr. M. — a man of 51. Murphy will probably inform Lawson when he arrives, but have Lawson inquire for Mr. M. at the front office of the P.B.B.H. each day so as to be sure he is not missed. This opportunity of having three new cases together is unique. Get without fail reticulocyte counts every day. If Lawson can guarantee to get a measured diet into Mr. M., I could have Mr. M. go to the Huntington if he could get a private room at not over $42 a week. Let him tell me his decision on Wednesday A.M. I hope to get to the H.M.H. by 10:30 A.M.

On Saturday morning, April 2, 1927, the Interurban Club met at the Children's Hospital, and George presented the results of the new work on "The Influence of Fractions of Liver on Pernicious Anemia." Mrs. B—— was the first patient to be treated with Fraction G, and since she had been longest under treatment, her case was important. George had all the data except the latest blood count, and Lawson was to get that before the lecture. Unfortunately, there was trouble with the solutions and Lawson did not reach the amphitheater until George had begun to speak. Lawson could see that George was uneasy, looking all around the room as he talked. Finally, however, Lawson in the back row caught his eye, and at once George interrupted himself: "Oh, there you are!" Everyone turned around to see who "you" was. George smiled, the audience tittered, and when Lawson came down to the floor of the amphitheater to add the latest figure to the copy of Mrs. B——'s chart on the blackboard, he got "a hand." When the figure showed the reticulocytes up to 41 percent, George was delighted and did not hide his satisfaction at this up-to-the-minute confirmation of his results.

This work on liver fractions was exciting. The whole staff of the Huntington, and many people at the Brigham, had caught George Minot's enthusiasm and were doing everything to help him. The importance of the discovery of liver was shown each day by the remarkable changes in the course of a disease which "only yesterday" had had a fatal outcome. The results were obvious — plainly evident for all to see. George Minot was more pleased than anyone. He was in good spirits when he and Marian came to dinner with us. "Rack, I seem to have started something that looks good," he said. "Do you by any chance have a little dividend in that shaker?"

After the meeting in Atlantic City, George's fame spread. Invitations to appear before medical societies of various sizes and importance came in. In February, he had six of these engagements ahead of him, and the data for two more papers were ready to be put together for publication. George wrote to Dr. Locke: "I had to refuse a swell chance to write for an English-edited book on Blood. It tears my heart out that neither of us can do it. We are just too crowded with other things." In another letter he asked, "Could we meet Sunday A.M. between 10 and 12:30? Every other second is hopelessly jammed up — it's terrific! — It isn't cases so much as the affairs of many people connected with the School and the Hospital." It was not easy to make three different institutions — the Huntington, the Cancer Commission, and the Harvard Medical School — all work together. At times it was hard to place responsibility, and to find the real authority.

A time-consuming business was that of answering the considerable correspondence that developed as soon as liver extract became available. Many doctors were asking: "What is the best preparation for my patient, and what is the dose?" "How long should the treatment be continued?" "What diet should be prescribed when the patient is taking liver by mouth or liver extract by injections?"

Each letter was answered carefully, but I have heard George say: "Goodness knows I have tried to describe the treatment in all its details as carefully as I can, and you must agree that you can find a good paper about it in many different journals. If the doctors would only read what is right there — right on their own desks, probably — they would not have to ask so many questions. I suppose it is easier to write a letter than to go to the library."

Private practice was another responsibility. It was a sort of necessary nuisance. Medical discoveries, even big ones, do not pay the landlord and the grocer, at least in the beginning.

George had his eye on two new men to help in the office and in the hospital — Dr. Francis T. Hunter and Dr. George P. Reynolds. Both were well-trained young doctors, and if they could move over to 311 they could carry on their own practices, if any, and at the same time help the Associates by taking preliminary histories and doing laboratory work, in return for office space and a small stipend. Dr. Hunter did not stay long — his own researches at the Massachusetts General Hospital needed more of his time — but Dr. Reynolds eventually became an Associate, too.

In one of his longhand scrawls to Dr. Locke, George wrote: "Will you plan to have all our patients after basals at 311 get food — crackers, milk, or orange juice. Thank you." For the measurement of the basal metabolic rate the patient must be tested in the morning on an empty stomach before breakfast, and several patients had felt faint before leaving the office. Even without diabetes, George himself would have felt quite bad if under these conditions he could not have had his breakfast on time, and he had not a little sympathy for those who complained.

Dr. Locke's reply was short: "I am not sure that running a restaurant is a wise procedure, and I should like to consider it carefully with you and Jerry before taking the step." The matter was postponed.

In March 1927, when George had complained about the management of the office, Dr. Locke wrote him a friendly letter. Just why Minot and Locke had to write each other so many letters when they were so closely associated in their business is hard to say, except perhaps that George "liked to have it in writing." Here is a part of what Locke wrote:

> It is the greatest possible satisfaction to me to see the recognition which you are receiving. Your indefatigable spirit, your imagination, your big vision, your intense interest in team play just make the thing go. I simply could not keep the machine going without those contributions on your part. On the other side of the picture, however, is the fact that the machine has made your development possible. I think it is not an exaggeration to say that your career has to a very considerable degree been the direct result of the organization which has placed in your hands the effective tools.

In the year following the first announcement of the effect of liver in pernicious anemia, George Minot's fame had spread widely. On May 19, 1927, at the Annual Meeting of the American Medical Association held in Washington, D.C., the important paper on the morning program of the Section on Practice of Medicine was the report by Minot and Murphy entitled "A Diet Rich in Liver in the Treatment of Pernicious Anemia." [5]

Word about the importance of this paper had spread, and in the brief interval before it the members crowded in so that even the big ballroom of the Mayflower Hotel was packed with men. When the Chairman of the Section, our friend Dr. Rollin T. Woodyatt, introduced George, the entire audience rose to its feet and applauded as George walked forward to the rostrum.

Medical audiences do not do this often, but this time the admiration for Dr. George Minot and the appreciation of his achievement were so intense that they had to burst out spontaneously. Dr.

Arthur W. Allen, surgeon of Boston and a great friend, had come over from the surgical section of the meeting to hear the paper and was most impressed by the great reception that George was given. He recalls clearly the dignified, reserved, scholarly presentation that George made, the close attention that the audience gave to it, and then the enthusiastic, prolonged applause at the end. The number of cases treated with liver had increased from 45 in the original report to 105 in this second report, and all but 6 of them had done very well. Three of the six had not followed the diet as advised; the other three had died of causes not due to anemia. George was well pleased with the results of his treatment.

When he and Marian got home to Boston, he did not say much about the meeting except that it had been "successful." It was through others that I learned about the acclaim with which he had been greeted. He went back to work the next day.

He went to Maine for the summer, and on August 24, 1927, he wrote to Locke from Northeast Harbor:

> Dr. Best [Charles H. Best of Banting and Best] was here yesterday: delightful person: we talked for three hours . . .
>
> I have had a very fine letter from Sir T. Houston of Belfast, Ireland [which tells of his] remarkable results with the liver diet, and I have an invitation to address next May the Royal Society of Medicine in London. I think I should seriously consider going over and learning about medicine in England. I will want your views on this: I believe that Dr. E.P.J. [Joslin] considers I can go "O.K." and Best said: "Of course you can go." Furthermore, the President of the University of Chicago asks me to be one of two to give addresses at the opening of their new buildings on October 31 — Very Swell, etc., but I have promised to give the Newbold Lecture in Philadelphia on November 1, so I must refuse Chicago. Then comes an invite to speak in New York — but I shall refuse that too. I have a dozen English letters to answer.

On the fourth page of this same letter is this:

> I seem to have more than ever the urge to study and advance medicine and only wish I controlled in part a bigger clinic to adequately advance knowledge about blood and diet and to get a crew of younger people going intensively on the cancer problem. Banting, so Best tells me, is at that problem . . . along the lines already formulated for the Huntington — i.e. to follow up Burrowes' work and get a growth inhibiting factor comparable to the growth stimulator of liver.

I myself am pretty good. Tired plus when I got here but by and large pretty decent. Slight gastric discomfort at times. I dread the mass of duties and things I want to see done ahead. However, it's the old story.

The meeting of the Medical Exchange Club on November 21, 1927 was held in Cousin Jim's house at 188 Marlborough Street. George told us a number of interesting items about *pernicious anemia,* most of which he had learned since the Announcement in Atlantic City. Here are the notes:

1. The name "Pernicious Anemia" developed from an editorial in an English Medical Journal which commented upon Thomas Addison's original description in his monograph published in 1855. Now the Englishmen are going back to the original term of "Addison's Anemia."

2. The treatment with liver and liver extract is very successful. Since using it, no deaths have occurred from anemia alone; only from complications. The nerve symptoms do not improve with the diet, but they do not seem to progress. Other forms of anemia do not yield to the diet.

3. Relapses have occurred after omitting the liver diet which seems to be specific for the disease. Infections and other complications in general prevent any rapid improvement and are often responsible for the relapse.

4. Liver seems to stimulate the marrow specifically. The blood picture, crowded with large cells, rapidly changes to normal. In the later relapse, the treatment seems to be just as effective as it was in the first. Unusual and exceptional cases present problems.

5. One patient who had had over forty transfusions responded to the liver diet very slowly, perhaps because of an injury to the marrow by these transfusions. Another patient who had had her spleen out likewise was slow to respond, again perhaps because of bone marrow injury after the transfusions which she had had. Infections such as pyelitis and tuberculosis or disturbances like gall stones offer difficulties.

6. There are cases with apparently typical symptoms including achylia [lack of acid in the stomach] which are not severe, but they also improve by diet and are thereby prevented from developing any severe anemia. Older people improve more slowly. Since the disease does occur in families, it is well to look at other members to see if they, too, have achylia.

7. Patients with pernicious anemia have white hair and blue eyes. Five cases have on improvement had their hair turn brown again. Skin lesions are not unusual — a slight eczema — a dermatitis — perhaps only a dryness. Perhaps they, too, represent the same dietary deficiency.

8. Eosinophile cells up to 30 percent of the total white cells in the peripheral blood occasionally follow prolonged feeding of raw liver or

of cooked liver. (There is no difference in effect between raw and cooked liver.) The persistence of these eosinophile cells has in two or three cases preceded a drop in the red count for some unexplained reason.

9. Other factors in the diet have been studied. Fats make little difference. Extra vitamins are not helpful. Whipple's "Standard" dogs which are repeatedly bled to a standard low red count have been fed liver fractions and have shown a slight gain in red cells, but usually liver is not effective in secondary anemia. Two cases with a myeloblastoma [a tumor of the bone marrow] infiltrating most of the organs were regarded at first as two cases of "Pernicious Anemia." Neither of them responded to liver. One of them did have free acid in his stomach and the proper diagnosis should have been made.

10. Yeast cures pellagra [which is due to a deficiency of Vitamin B] — but it has no effect on pernicious anemia.

11. The nature of the active substance remains unknown. The "fraction" which Dr. Cohn has isolated is a small polypeptid and has a nitrogenous base. It is not Vitamin B. This latter has no effect. [We know today that the active principle is Vitamin B_{12} — a tiny fraction of the whole Vitamin B.] The fraction is effective in a dose of four grams a day. It will be available to the public on January 1, 1928. On it, more than eighty patients have shown striking improvement.

12. The effect of liver is shown by the reticulated red cells which rise sharply within three to eight days. The height to which they rise is inversely proportional to the red blood count. The lower the red count the faster the start. When the red count is about three million, the response in reticulated cells is low.

13. There is often a transient drop in the red count at the start of treatment. If the curve of reticulocytes is plotted in the red count curve, it is evident that at first all the increase in red cells is due to reticulocytes. The transient drop occurs early and before the reticulocytes have started.

14. When drawn blood containing numbers of reticulocytes is incubated, it will in a few hours show a loss of these young cells and when "fraction" is added *in vitro*, the loss of reticulum is very rapid as compared with controls; the cells become "mature." This obviously gives a test-tube method of estimating the potency of "fraction." Where liver is fed in or after a spontaneous remission, the rise in reticulated cells is far less striking.

The speed with which new discoveries in medicine are developed is amazing. It is amazing also to see how close some earlier investigator came to making the same discovery. A little later, George was inquisitive enough to spend more time in looking over the old literature to see what he could find about the relation between diet and anemia. The notes that he made in pencil for the Alvarez Lecture, which he gave in 1936, cover about 25 pages of yellow block — some of them in Marian's writing as George dictated. They include three paragraphs:

> A prophetic statement was made by Austin Flint in 1860 when he wrote: "Nor is it difficult to see how fatal anemia must follow an amount of degenerative disease reducing the amount of gastric juice so far that the assimilation of food is rendered wholly inadequate to the wants of the body."
>
> In 1870 Samuel Fenwick wrote a paper in the *Lancet* on "Atrophy of the Stomach." [6] He described a typical case of pernicious anemia in which the secreting tubules of the stomach were atrophied into a mass of connective tissue. He showed that pepsin was absent, and he wrote that the progressive atrophy of the stomach had prevented the digestion of the albuminous material of the food. Apparently, he had consided that this was the cause of anemia, and added, "Perhaps future investigators may prove that the anemia arises from a co-existing atrophy of the stomach or other parts of the digestive canal."
>
> In subsequent papers, and in his book[7] published ten years later in 1880, Fenwick records further distinctive observations and remarks concerning the relation of the blood to the state of the digestive tract. There were other studies concerning the stomach in pernicious anemia, but none so significant as Fenwick's study. There are references, also, to the relationship between the gastro-intestinal tract and iron deficiency anemias, especially chlorosis. There was a waxing and waning interest in this subject until 1928, when Castle subjected his brilliant original ideas to experiment and proved the important role of a factor secreted by the normal stomach.

In the *Archives of Internal Medicine* for July 1923 — and that was three years before George's announcement — is the paper by Drs. R. B. Gibson and Campbell P. Howard from the Research Laboratory of the Iowa State University which George referred to in his original communication. In their "Metabolic Studies in Pernicious Anemia," [8] Gibson and Howard investigated the metabolism of fats and of nitrogen, and their third object was "to test the efficiency of Whipple's high iron diet when given to patients suffering from 'idiopathic anemia.'" They observed that "more favorable nitrogen, and especially iron, balances may be readily established in pernicious anemia when diets rich in food iron (Whipple) and comparatively low in caloric and protein values are given," but their paper says nothing about liver.

Iron was always important to George, and his notes on chlorosis are interesting. Hypochromic anemia (chlorosis) was common in young women in their twenties, and he wondered why it should occur at this particular time of life. He recognized that the girls have depraved appetites and explained that a vicious circle becomes established easily: improper food — deficient iron intake — anemia — poor health — poor appetite — less food — less iron —more anemia — more poor health — and so on until at last proper feeding and management can be effected and the chain can be broken.

George found out that in 1895 Stockman[9] had written a sound, but little appreciated, critical treatise on chlorosis in which he described two direct causes. One was blood loss — with menstruation — and the other was an insufficient intake of iron. George explained that it takes about 3 milligrams of iron to make 10 grams of hemoglobin, and the daily requirement of iron is about 5 milligrams a day. Infections, stomach disturbances, and menstruation all affect the intake. Stockman noted that the need for iron increases rapidly in females between the ages of fourteen and eighteen, when the growth is rapid, and that at this time the need is more than doubled. If the stomach lacks acid, the appetite is even poorer, and the blood loss by menses is even greater. One must keep in mind the initial cause, the contributing cause, and then the added causes, which result "viciously" from the disease itself.

For Christmas that year, George sent me a book, and with it a note:

> The botany book — Millspaugh's *Medicinal Plants*[10] — I send because the plates are rather nice and because asthma experts should know the "beasts" from which the pollens come . . .
>
> It is interesting to realize that 100 ± years ago the medical schools gave a full course in medical botany — it was apparently a major subject, and Jacob Bigelow wrote a treatise thereon. And by the way, do you know why the name of Gardenia was given that excellent white perfumed flower? It was because Linnaeus named it such after Dr. Gardener of Charleston, S.C., who lived about 1730 and was a famous M.D. of the time . . . His fame was particularly through his advance in knowledge concerning medical botany.*

* In the *New England Journal of Medicine 253,* 610 (October 6, 1955) is a paper by Dr. Andrew Kerr, Jr., of New Orleans. Interested in medical history, he found that Dr. Alexander Garden (1728–1793), a physician who was also a naturalist, migrated to Charleston, South Carolina, where he regretted that "there is not a living soul who

Where did George find time to browse through old books when he was so harassed with "forty-eleven things to do"? His inquisitiveness and his broad interests enabled him to use his periods of relaxation with profit to make his interests still broader.

One of the things that George had been thinking about and talking about was "What is going to happen to the Thorndike?" The next chapter tells.

---

knows the least iota of Natural History." Dr. Garden corresponded with his teacher, Carl Linnaeus of Upsala, sending specimens of both plants and animals to him. In the twelfth edition of his *Systema Naturae* (1767) Linnaeus gives Garden credit for describing several new genera of both plants and fishes. Dr. Kerr writes: "To honor this 'happy illustrator of Nature of Carolina' Linnaeus named, in 1762, a spectacular ornamental shrub 'Gardenia' [even though] Garden did not describe the plant."

9

The Thorndike Memorial Laboratory

George Minot had always had great admiration and respect for Francis Weld Peabody. The decision to enter the Medical School in the beginning was encouraged by Peabody's talks. The desire to become an intern at the Massachusetts General Hospital and then to work with Dr. Thayer in Baltimore had been fostered by Peabody's accounts of his own activities. George recognized Francis as a superior person with a remarkably broad outlook on life. Francis had been one of the first to see the changes in medicine that were coming. He had read the Flexner Report, and he had discussed it with George enthusiastically.

George was always impressed by Francis' manifold experiences, his travels, and the series of interesting and important positions that he had held. George himself would not have gone to study chemistry under Professor Emil Fischer in Berlin nor to work under Professor August Krogh or Professor Sörenson in Copenhagen as Francis did; he would not have liked to be so far away from home. Francis had been the first Resident Physician when the Hospital of the Rockefeller Institute for Medical Research in New York was opened in 1910, and in 1913, he became the first Resident Physician at the Peter Bent Brigham Hospital in Boston. Still later, he was a member of the Rockefeller Commission to establish a medical school in China, traveling through Europe and across Russia. During the war he had gone with the Red Cross to Rumania, making another trip on the Trans-Siberian Railway to reach Rumania by the "back door."

In 1918, as a major in the Army, he was put in charge of the cardiovascular unit at Lakewood, New Jersey. At about that time, George Minot was engaged in his trinitrotoluene studies, and was staying with Dorothy and me at Englewood. I was on duty at Camp Merritt nearby. George and I drove over to Lakewood one afternoon, and heard a little about Peabody's travels. During his tour of duty at Lakewood, he did much to unravel the mysteries of the "effort syndrome," sometimes called "irritable heart" or "neurocirculatory asthenia," demonstrating that the rapid pulse rates and high blood pressures disappeared as soon as the patients were released from the service.[1] A little later, Peabody was medical consultant in France, where the vast activities of the American Army impressed him greatly.

After the war, it was at the Huntington that George came into professional as well as personal contact with Francis Peabody, and after that Francis' influence on George was even stronger. Francis was married at that time (1919), and George and Marian met the Peabodys often. Both Marian Minot and Virginia Peabody had the ability to arrange social gatherings that were successful and purposeful, with people whose talk was both pleasant and instructive to them and to their husbands.

In 1919, new buildings and new laboratories were going up in most of the medical schools all over the country. New professorships of medicine were being created. Francis Peabody had become a noted member of the medical profession, and he received several invitations to become Professor of Medicine, each invitation more tempting than the last. Fortunately, he declined them all, for in the spring of 1921 the Trustees of the Boston City Hospital gave him the opportunity of setting up and directing a new Department of Research, which was to be established in a new building to be provided by a bequest. Mr. George L. Thorndike (1847–1901) was a lawyer who had left money to the Boston City Hospital in order to erect a memorial building in honor of his brother, Dr. William H. Thorndike (1824–1884), a well-known general practitioner in Boston.

Here, then, was some of the money to carry out a plan that Dr. Peabody had always cherished, and he accepted the position with pleasure. He persuaded the trustees that the responsibility of the Boston City Hospital was not limited to the care and treatment of individual patients, but included medical teaching, preventive medicine, and medical research. He pointed out first, that good treatment of the patients depends upon careful study of their problems; second, that this study is more careful if it is made for two purposes — to learn more about the disease, and to teach the students about it; and third, that no teacher or professor will spend much of his time and effort in the public wards of a hospital unless by doing so he will add to his own knowledge and experience. It is easy to see that the best students and the best doctors will find their way to those institutions and to those positions in which they will have opportunities to learn and to improve their own education and their experience.

The trustees had heard about this before. They had had requests for small appropriations with which to buy laboratory supplies, and they had heard talk about salaries for doctors to work on a full-time basis, but until Francis Peabody could confirm so eloquently the previous urgings of such men as Dr. Edwin A. Locke and Dr. George G. Sears, they had been quite skeptical about the propriety of using the public's money for research. This time, however, they listened and they approved. In April 1921, the City Hospital Trustees authorized a loan appropriation of $150,000 to supplement Mr. Thorndike's bequest. The four-story building cost $313,000 and took two full years to build.

In the fall of 1921, the Peking Union Medical College was completed, and Dr. Peabody, taking his wife with him, made his third trip to China, this time to take part in the dedication and to stay on as professor until the medical service could be well established.

When he came back in February 1922, his headquarters were still at the Brigham, but his thoughts were mostly at the Boston City Hospital. The construction of the Thorndike was interesting, but the selection of personnel to work in the new place was more interesting, and what should go on inside when the building was ready was the most interesting problem of all. How his new laboratory should dovetail into the workings of the enormous City Hospital was a question that led him to think and to talk and to write about "The Function of a Municipal Hospital" [2] and the reasons why the good students are not attracted to these large public institutions. The answer was not hard to find. Not only was the staff worn down by the enormous routine, but there were neither opportunities nor facilities for making chemical analyses or physical measurements which might show whether some new and interesting idea was any good or not. A teaching hospital is a good hospital, because the students are there to ask questions and thereby to stimulate the doctor-teacher. Improvement in care and treatment follows immediately whenever the patient and his case can be studied and discussed thoroughly. "The fostering of research is one of the most important means of enabling a hospital to perform its full functions," Dr. Peabody said, "and it is of great significance that the Trustees of the Boston City Hospital have established a complete Division of Medical Research in the Thorndike Memorial Laboratory." The Thorndike was to become a unique institution, unique in part because of the atmosphere that Francis Peabody established in it.

It was in August 1923 that the staff began to move their equipment into the new laboratories, but it was not until November that the Thorndike Ward was opened for patients. Three years later, George Minot was to read his paper — The Paper — in Atlantic City. As Secretary of the Association of American Physicians, Francis was sitting on the platform behind the rostrum on that memorable occasion; he was one of the first to congratulate George.

During the summer of 1926, both George and Francis were on vacation in Northeast Harbor, Maine. This time Francis was not well. He had been having indigestion, and he had been losing weight. George Minot saw him almost daily, and then finally, in July, Francis went to Boston for a complete examination. The results were quite unsuspected, and they were shocking to everybody, for the x-ray examination showed a large tumor in the wall of the stomach, and at operation it was found to be impossible to take the tumor out. On August 6, Francis went back to Northeast Harbor, and Dr. Locke wrote to George:

> Francis leaves today. Everyone here is completely stunned. Zinsser, Drinker, and others have broken down and cried after they have seen him. Edsall will feel it keenly, of course. I am to dine with him next week. With Francis there in Northeast, it will be hard for you in some ways, but you should feel happy to be in a position to mean so much to Francis.

On August 23, George wrote to me:

> I meant to get some work done up here, but not a stroke so far. Peabo and wife dined here tonight — all so natural. He actually looks better

than a week ago. It has been a pleasant natural evening, and now that he has gone it seems uncanny, unbelievable, to realize what there is within him. Miracles have occurred: we only hope that others may occur. When I return is a puzzle. It has become clear that Wearn or I are to be here as long as Peabo is — probably till about September 15.

In the next January, Francis Peabody gave at the Harvard Medical School one of the Sunday afternoon series of public lectures on "The Care of the Patient." [3] Only a few days before he died, he remarked to his wife, "You know, I have an idea that the writing of that talk was the best thing I ever did!" Today, twenty-nine years later, the things that this little book says are just as new, just as vital, and just as true as they were on that Sunday afternoon in January 1927. Every student and every doctor should keep his copy within reach of his desk chair. The last paragraph is the summary that is so familiar to all good doctors. It bears repeating once again:

> One of the essential qualities of the clinician is interest in humanity, for the secret of the care *of* the patient is in caring *for* the patient.

In the spring of 1927, Francis Peabody was still carrying on in the face of a dreadful disease. I remember seeing him sitting in a steamer chair in his garden in Cambridge on a lovely day in the spring. He stood up to greet me and was full of interest in what I was doing — wanted to know all about the study of asthma and what was going on in the clinic and in the laboratory. He asked a number of questions, and made several suggestions, which indicated that he was quite familiar with some of the newer advances in the study of the problem; he had been reading as usual. George, of course, saw him quite regularly, and came back with a similar report: "Rack, it is remarkable the way that man carries on. I bet he is uncomfortable, but he is cheerful and his mind is just as clear as ever."

During that summer of 1927, Francis Peabody was not strong enough to go to Maine. His wife agreed with the doctors that it would be safer and easier for all if he stayed in Cambridge.

A letter came from his friend, Dr. Warfield T. Longcope, who by that time had moved from New York to become Professor of Medicine at Johns Hopkins:

Dear Francis,

There must be something in all of us which makes us want to be physicians rather than pure scientists; and I am sure that the thing ["The Care of the Patient"] which you have so highly developed and have given . . . to all of us, is far more important for the clinic than experimental research . . . Is it possible for the Head of the clinic to develop it to the highest extent and at the same time to make important contributions to science? You have come nearer to it than anyone else . . . Nobody has formulated it as you have. None of us has been quite so conscious of it before, and we must all strive to put this into the clinics so that we may develop better clinicians and better scientists, and not turn out machines that grind out cold, spiritless facts.

This letter seemed to provide a "fresh renewal of intellectual energy" as the *Memoir*[4] has it, and it led Dr. Peabody to dictate a reply that covered sixteen pages. This reply was such an important document that it was published after his death as a special article, under the title "The Soul of the Clinic." [5]

George Minot appreciated the paper as a sort of summary or statement of what he knew already, and later it became a guide to his own policy and behavior. Dr. Peabody had no desire to make all clinics conform to the same pattern — the different circumstances under which they operated demanded different treatment — but certain essentials were the same.

The man at the head is the Important Person, for he sets the atmosphere. The selection of this Chief is therefore of fundamental consequence, and the paper discusses it:

When a professorship falls open, the committee in charge . . . usually says somewhat naïvely that it is looking for a man who has had an intensive scientific training, has done important research, is a good administrator, is a competent teacher, and finally has had clinical experience . . . Such a man is, of course, almost impossible to find. "Clinical experience" is apt to be put last among the specifications. This is because some of our friends think that clinical medicine can be "picked up" very easily by the prospective professor . . . We know that clinical medicine is a subject which is to be mastered only by years of long, hard experience and if any of the members of the committee to select a professor were taken sick . . . I am pretty certain they would rate "experience" higher [than technical knowledge]. The argument . . . that someone else can tell the students how to take care of patients is . . . beside the point, because it begins by accepting as insignificant what is a very important function of the department.

The paper describes the general ward as the backbone of the clinic, and it shows why the relation of the Chief to the ward should be real and not fictitious. "Standards of thought as well as of action are set from above . . . The dignity [of the ward] becomes impaired . . . just as soon as the chief separates himself from it."

After saying that "research is a type of training which develops critical judgment" and that "the younger members of the staff should all take part in some research problem," Dr. Peabody emphasizes the dominant position of the Chief and his many responsibilities toward all the members of his staff, including the direction and supervision of the young men doing research. The Chief is, of course, "harassed by forty-eleven things to do," as George Minot would say, and Dr. Peabody is well aware of this important problem:

> One frequently hears it said that if the chief is a good administrator, he will divide all this work up and put it on the shoulders of his assistants. To a certain extent this [division of his work] is possible . . . but experience has shown me that . . . the major part of the responsibility must be assumed by the chief.

The next sentences reveal his warm regard for his fellow men.

> It is not only to these dignitaries [heads of departments] that the chief must leave his door ajar . . . How often one finds interns and students lurking outside. "Can I have five minutes with you, Sir?" You let him in, sit down and find that what he has approached so modestly is the problem of his whole career . . . Is there on the whole anything more important than giving advice about a young man's life?

In discussing the differences between full-time and part-time teachers, he says, "Men who are in outside practice have something to contribute but private patients are important . . . They are . . . the cases that stick in my mind . . . The main point is that the patient has sought you or me personally and not the hospital." The paper ends with this excellent line, written only a day or two before his death:

"What we want is less of the system and law that kills and more of the spirit that gives life."

On October 13, 1927, Francis Peabody died at the very prime of his life, at the age of forty-six. Everyone connected with the Harvard Medical School suffered a direct personal loss, and George Minot suffered more than the others. Not only had George lost a close friend, but he had lost a wise mentor to whom he had always been able to look for counsel and support.

For the Medical School and the Thorndike Memorial Laboratory, the loss was a serious matter in another way. The development of their laboratory was likely to slow down, and Peabody's plans for the future might not be carried out. Where could the Medical School Faculty find a man who would take over Francis Peabody's ideals and his leadership? The Faculty discussed the matter at some length and concluded that there was only one really good candidate —George Richards Minot.

On January 21, 1928, George wrote me a very interesting letter on a piece of yellow block:

> I suppose . . . that the birds have gossiped with you in these past 10 weeks while my mind has been tormented to be able to talk it all over with you. Laying plans to totally change one's career [is a] large order, and to be even thought of for the highest sort of medical position in America is beyond my comprehension. I am overcome with the honor. How I can ever come within miles of serving American Medicine and our School as Francis did, I do not know. I am ordered to try, and they know all my faults. It's an ordeal and a pleasure, but seems colossal for a little mite to do. Hold your tongue — until I can talk with you on Monday.

This letter was written to me as an intimate friend. George's humility was real; it was not affected. He had, of course, known that he was being considered for the appointment, for the Committee had to sound him out to see whether he would be willing to move from the Huntington to the Thorndike in case he was elected. The Committee found that he was not only willing but anxious to go. His humility resulted from his understanding of the responsibilities, as well as the opportunities, before him.

On April 1, 1928, Dr. George R. Minot, then aged forty-two, resigned his position as Chief of the Medical Service at the Huntington Memorial Hospital to become Director of the Thorndike Memorial Laboratory at the Boston City Hospital. Dr. Joseph C. Aub was appointed to take his place at the Huntington. With this move, recognition of George increased. His title in the Medical School was changed from "Clinical Professor of Medicine," a limited appointment, to "Professor of Medicine," an appointment "without limit of time."

When George Minot entered the Thorndike in the spring of 1928, he knew what Dr. Peabody's paper, "The Soul of the Clinic," had told him: that after this his job was to teach young men, and that the hours when he could look through the microscope or do any investigative work on his own would be few and far between.

At the Thorndike, a number of important researches were in their very active stages, and a number of men destined to become important in American medicine were working there.

Dr. Hermann L. Blumgart had come with Dr. Peabody from the Brigham. His interest in blood flow had been intensified by his contact with Dr. Cecil K. Drinker and he was working on the ingenious idea of injecting a solution of a radioactive salt into the arm vein on one side and then detecting the time of its arrival in the other arm by an apparatus called a Wilson cloud chamber. (The Geiger counter came later.) After Dr. Minot became Director, Dr. Blumgart stayed on for a few months and then became the first of the Thorndike staff to be called to an important position. He went to the new Beth Israel Hospital in Boston, where a little later he became Chief of the Medical Staff.

In Dr. Peabody's second year at the Thorndike (1925) two very important men were added to his staff. The first was Dr. Soma Weiss. Born in Hungary, Weiss graduated M.D. from Columbia College of Physicians and Surgeons in New York in 1923. He was a very attractive man as well as an extraordinary student, who developed and retained an amazing grasp of medical literature. During his internship at Bellevue Hospital in New York City, he had demonstrated his own particular inquisitiveness. He had come upon a patient with a rare and remarkable disorder. Since the patient said that he had been in the hospital of Edinburgh University, Dr. Weiss realized that he had probably been seen by a certain clinician whom Dr. Weiss remembered as the author of a paper on that particular disease. If so, the clinician had probably reported the case. Sure enough, the index in the library led Dr. Weiss to the paper in which the Scottish doctor had described the early study of a patient with the same initials as the present patient. Dr. Eugene F. Dubois, Chief of the Service at Bellevue, was delighted with the enterprise of his young intern. George liked to tell how he met Soma Weiss one afternoon in June 1925, at Northeast Harbor, where Weiss was staying in Dr. Peabody's house. He was fascinated by the Hungarian accent, as well as by his beautiful use of the English language.

At the Thorndike in 1925, Dr. Weiss worked at first with Dr. Blumgart. Together they simplified the problem of measuring the velocity of blood flow. When ether is injected into the arm vein — a small dose given rapidly — the time when the taste or smell of ether appears is another measure of the velocity — the "arm-to-tongue" time. In 1927 Blumgart and Weiss[6] used histamine, a cholinergic substance concerned with the regulation of local blood supply. The time when the flushing of the face and the sense of warmth develops after the intravenous injection serves as another index of the speed of blood flow and that bit of research led to other studies of histamine — Weiss was a pharmacologist — which became very important. Soma Weiss worked at the Thorndike for fourteen years, and during that time his name appeared on 150 papers, concerned mostly with the heart and the arteries. In 1935 one of his observations was concerned with the carotid sinus reflex. He had observed that in certain individuals pressure with the finger on a particular spot on the neck causes fainting. With Dr. Eugene B. Ferris, Jr., and Dr. Richard B. Capps,[7] he showed that in man it is the carotid sinus, a small island of nerve tissue in the wall of the big carotid artery, and not the brain which is sensitive to a lowering of the oxygen "pressure" in the blood. When oxygen is deficient, as at high altitude, it is the carotid sinus which sends a message to the respiratory center in the brain to increase the breathing. In our ordinary daily life, however, the depth and frequency of our breathing is controlled by the respiratory center itself — a group of cells which is sensitive to the accumulation of carbon dioxide (CO_2) in the blood; the increase in CO_2 after exercise makes the blood more acid, and this acid stimulates the brain.

Dr. William Bosworth Castle was the second important man added to Dr. Peabody's staff. He also came to the Thorndike in 1925. He was a classmate of Dr. Blumgart in the Harvard Medical School (1921), and had taken his internship at the Massachusetts General Hospital. He, too, had been guided and stimulated in his student days by Dr. Cecil K. Drinker. During two years at the Harvard School of Public Health, he had worked with Drinker on problems concerned with the physiology of digestion and blood formation. At the Thorndike, his interest centered promptly on the observation that patients with pernicious anemia have no acid in their stomachs, and he asked himself, "What does that mean?" It was not long before he made the first of those remarkable experiments with gastric juice which were to show that in pernicious anemia the stomach is deficient in something besides acid, and that the "something" is the "intrinsic factor." At that time he thought of this as a property of normal stomach juice which can digest protein food to "make" the special active principle so necessary for the proper nourishment of the bone marrow. We know now that this principle is vitamin B_{12}. The feeding of liver is effective because liver contains so much of the B_{12} that some of it can be absorbed directly and without the need to "make" it with the help of the missing enzymelike "intrinsic factor."

Dr. Joseph T. Wearn had come with Dr. Peabody from the Brigham to the Thorndike. The research under his direction was concerned with the blood supply to the heart muscle. He showed [8] that in the heart, as in other tissues, the capillary network of blood vessels is elastic. Its various parts are interchangeable: the capillaries can open or close in accordance with the need for greater or less blood in that area. When the heart must beat 24 hours a day, it is a clever arrangement to have different blood vessels, and probably different muscle fibers, become active and inactive by turns. There are times when some of them can rest, and there are other times when all of them must work together.

When Dr. George Minot took charge of the Thorndike he found that Dr. Peabody had left behind very much of a going concern.

In the modern teaching hospital work on new problems — on researches — such as those just described is only one activity of the postgraduate student. True it is that his achievements in the laboratory or his studies on the ward constitute a large measure of his success and determine his advancement in the field of academic medicine, but it is also true that his job is to take care of the patients assigned to him and to supervise the young undergraduate students in his service, whether on the wards or in the out-patient department, or perhaps in the two places on different days. The selection and presentation of interesting patients before classes, large or small, at which the Chief will preside is often another duty.

George and I were talking about this one night. "You know," he said, "one must be careful that this research business is not overdone. I put it this way: It is easy to get so involved in one's research problems that one forgets about medicine as a whole. The residents don't like to work in the general medical out-patient department, and not all of them care too much about spending time at the bedside; their research seems to them so much more important. I am sure, however, that it is essential that every doctor, regardless of his particular field of interest, should keep his hands on patients, and we must help him to become a well-rounded, well-trained physician."

At his first staff conference in the Thorndike, George was a little uneasy. He wanted to make a good impression. He realized that he was in contact with men who were mature and who had already made their mark. He knew instinctively that they were studying him, anxious to see what changes he might suggest. He sat very straight in his chair, his sharp features sharper than ever, the lines in his face deeper. He was tense and a bit excited, but he saw at once that the men respected him and had confidence in his ability to guide them, and this thought restored his equanimity. He said, "This is a good laboratory, not so much because of its excellent equipment as because of the opportunities for freedom of thought and for open discussion which Francis Peabody established. Each of you knows much more about your own problems than I do, and I cannot help you directly, but I will try to maintain what I like to call the 'atmosphere' which is such an important asset to this laboratory."

In March 1928, George gave one of the "Harvey Lectures" [9] in New York. This was an important assignment. The Harvey Society invited only the best — the top men — to come to them, and the invitation was an honor as well as an obligation. In an excellent lecture, George reviewed the work on pernicious anemia and its treatment.

In May 1928, he was sick with a respiratory infection and could not go to the annual meeting of the Association of American Physicians in Atlantic City. At that meeting he was chosen to receive the Kober Medal for 1929. This medal is awarded annually to "a member of the Association of American Physicians who has contributed to the progress and achievements of the medical sciences or preventive medicine." It was a real honor, and it pleased George, as it pleased all his friends. I sent him a telegram, which he acknowledged on a printed commercial postcard, redirected to me: "Your telegram brought me news that is embarrassing. They certainly have conferred an honor on me."

In June came a letter to me, written in longhand, and on George's new Thorndike stationery: "One likes to have his most intimate friend . . . hear news at first hand. The University appears to wish to do me an honor on Commencement day (five days hence), and I am informed that President Lowell is to hand me a parchment to hang on the wall and enable me to write D.Sc. after my name besides A.B. and M.D. I dine with the President on Wed. Eve."

The extra words in the letter are not silly. They were George's way of showing his great satisfaction. He was not boasting, and he knew that I, too, would be pleased. President Lowell's citation, read at the Harvard Commencement, June 21, 1928, reads: "George Richards Minot, Doctor of Science, a medical explorer who has abolished a fatal malady and opened a road for more recovery."

In the fall of 1928, after his return from Northeast Harbor, George started the new academic year. New men had been selected with great care, and he was pleased that they were coming to work in his department as Assistant Resident Physicians. Dr. Maxwell Finland, Dr. Laurence B. Ellis, and Dr. Clark Heath had been classmates in Harvard Medical School Class of 1916, and now they had completed their internships. Each was a well-trained young man, and each had appealed to George as being a person who was likely to succeed in medicine. To each man George had explained the "system" — how he would be left alone to pursue his problem in his own way, and that about once a month he would be expected to present at the Staff Conference his new observations and ideas. The patients on the Second and Fourth — the Harvard — Services of the Boston City Hospital were close by, and Assistant Residents in the Thorndike were expected to keep their eyes on the wards in order to recognize interesting patients, and perhaps to find a key case to be studied carefully. As soon as a patient was transferred to the Thorndike ward for special study and treatment, one of the Residents took full responsibility for every detail of his care.

George gave occasional lectures, or conferences, to the Harvard Medical students in the Thorndike Amphitheater. At first the audience was small, but as George's fame spread more men came to hear him. The lectures were prepared carefully, and they were distinctly formal. On lecture days George chose the right necktie and wore the right suit, so as to make the right appearance. He was not an easy talker. He tried at times to include a little levity, but the effect was not very successful.

Conferences with the Thorndike Staff were held on Wednesdays at noon, with the Assistants and the Residents gathered around the table in the library next door to George's office. Each time the conference would begin: "Gentlemen, today Dr. X will tell us what he has been doing." That was all; there was no special title for the introduction. Each man knew what his companion had been investigating, and here was a chance to learn the details, to ask questions, and to make suggestions. The idea was excellent. When the discussion was controlled and directed, each young investigator helped the others. Some of the discussions in these conferences were warm, if not actually heated. George would usually let them go, for the arguments made everyone think hard. Quite often he would sit there looking out of the window, not seeming to pay much attention.

One day, when the talk was almost too lively, he got up suddenly. "Look at that!" he exclaimed. "There are two blackbirds — no, they are starlings — sitting on that tree. I bet they are the same ones I saw the other day. Haven't seen any before for a year; where do they come from?"

Everybody's attention was diverted from the arguments; the men all laughed and left the conference in good humor. Each man could clarify his own thoughts on the problem and perhaps extend his observations in the laboratory so as to strengthen his side of the argument or else to find that the opposition was right after all. The principles of self-education must be encouraged and fostered. George reminded his men that they were working on the outer boundaries of knowledge, and they must learn that their progress depended on the active synthesis of their own thinking processes and not upon the passive absorption of facts discovered by others; the spoon-feeding era had passed long since.

There were several reasons why these conferences were successful. The first and foremost was that his men were good to start with. Dr. Minot had a genius for appraising their scientific ability, as well as their personal character. He wanted, and he obtained, men who were good students, to be sure, but also he wanted men who were attractive, bright, and cheerful, who had something to say for themselves, who had a high sense of integrity, and who were seeking the truth. The selection of his men was based partly on his own appraisal, but it was based more on what was learned from teachers and others who had known the man. Here, for example, is an interview which one of the candidates described to me many years later:

"When Dr. Minot was interviewing me for the position of Assistant Resident, he asked, 'What would you do if the door opened and a man about fifty years old came in and then fell forward flat on his face — unconscious?' I began to think to myself: 'The man tripped and in falling hit his head . . . He was a bit old for epilepsy — apoplexy is more likely . . . What causes cardiac standstill?' I was struggling to arrange my thoughts when Dr. Minot interrupted them:

" 'That is a tough situation, and when the bystander says "Get a doctor," it just might be you or me that would be called.' The idea seemed to interest him, and instead of waiting for me to give my answer, Dr. Minot went right ahead to illustrate the problem with a number of anecdotes. Then and there he taught me a good deal about this kind of emergency. The peculiar part was that he didn't let me talk at all; he didn't want to quiz me particularly, and I didn't have to say a word, but, you know, he seemed to know all about me anyway, and I got the appointment, all right."

I told him: "Of course Dr. Minot knew all about you. You may be sure that he had asked many others what they thought of you. The 'interview' was merely to check your appearance, your personality, and perhaps your manners, and to make sure that you were in fact the man he had in mind. He was honest with you and with himself when he just chatted."

The second reason for success was that George left his men alone.

He was not too concerned about the particular problem that any one man had chosen to study. If it interested the man, that was enough, and one could assume that the investigation would be interesting and profitable.

Third, there was the responsibility concerned with the expenditure of considerable sums of money for the support of these young men, as well as for the technicians and the apparatus and supplies for the laboratory in general. It was quite proper to require evidence of progress from time to time, and of achievement at the end. Incidentally, he wanted each piece of work finished promptly and not allowed to drag. "Button it up," he would say.

Teaching on the wards at the patient's bedside is the exercise that gives the teacher his greatest opportunity. By his attitude toward the patient, and by his ability to lead the discussion into the proper channels, he can be very effective. When the student presented his history to the group around the bed, George listened always with close attention.

"Where did you say he lived?"

"East Boston."

"Yes, I know, but what sort of a place is it? A single house or a small apartment? Sometimes we find five people living in four rooms, and I do not like that; I doubt if they do, either!

"Does any sunlight get into the place? What about noise, and what about smoke and dirt? What really interests me is his diet; please tell us all about that."

And, being Dr. Minot's student, he could tell "us" a good deal about it, and when the student had finished, the Professor asked still more details from the patient.

"Do you have meat?"

"Yes, Doctor."

"Do you eat meat?"

"No, Doctor."

"Gentlemen, you see now why it is that I have to be so fussy about words. It is very easy to be caught off guard, and particularly when the patient hesitates to confess that he has not been eating properly. Well, let's go on —" and he turned to the patient: "What time do you get home at night? When do you have dinner — and where? Does the whole family eat together?"

"No, I eat all alone while the others listen to the radio."

"Gentlemen, do you like that? I don't. My food would not taste good if there were noise and confusion and I was told to hurry up. Maybe that is one reason why this man has lost weight — what do you think?"

George wrote an "intercommunication" — on the back of an envelope — to Dr. Locke, Chief of the Fourth Service, who was visiting on the wards at that time: "I wish you would talk to your men about Rounds. They should begin on time. Also, it would help greatly if when I reached the ward the house officer could give me a list of the new cases that had been assigned to students and a list of the other new cases which had so far not been assigned. Also, I would like a list of the consultations that I am to see on other wards. With these lists, I can plan my time, and all of us will be better off."

Another note to Dr. Locke, this time on a piece torn out of a yellow block, says: "The number of doctors who come to see what we are doing is increasing. Should we form a committee to consider graduate teaching? Who will be responsible for it? We must consider our policies carefully." And he added: "Life is busy all right. Last week I was tired and weak as a rag, but today I am better."

In October there was talk about the International Physiological Congress scheduled for the summer of 1929: "What should we do about that? What part will the Thorndike play? It is not too early to be thinking about it."

In November he went to New York to give a lecture, and Marian went with him, of course. George wrote to Dr. Locke from the St. Regis Hotel: "We had a sumptuous meal last night at Pierre's; it was grossly expensive." George loved to eat good food in a "swell" place, and one can believe that he got his money's worth in pleasure, if not in calories. "I saw Jerry Blake in the distance, all smiles, evidentally enjoying himself, but when we met afterwards he, too, seemed to notice the cost of things in New York."

The first winter at the Thorndike was a busy and exciting time. There was reason to think that Soma Weiss would stay on at the Thorndike and rise to the position of Associate Director, which had been left vacant when Dr. Wearn was called to the Professorship of Medicine at Western Reserve University School of Medicine in Cleveland. George knew well that Weiss was good, and he was delighted that his promotion in the School and at the Thorndike could be arranged.

A little later Soma Weiss became very important to George. Soma would drop in to the Chief's office almost every morning for a chat, which was helpful to both George and himself. Dr. Weiss understood human nature so well that he could help greatly in solving many administrative problems, whether concerned with individuals or with general policies. If there was some trouble with the nursing service on the Thorndike Ward, or with a certain technician, it was Weiss who could approach the authorities with tact and a touch of humor, and they would soon agree that the situation was not right. George himself was so honest and so direct that his requests became almost demands, and when the City Hospital administration wanted to "think about it a little" — to discuss the matter before deciding on action — Dr. Minot was inclined to be just a trifle impatient about it. Dr. James W. Manary, at that time Superintendent of the City Hospital, has told me of his great admiration and respect for Dr. Minot — that he was "always a perfect gentleman" — but he implied that talks with Dr. Minot were not always easy.

In March 1929, George went to Baltimore to give the Thayer Lecture. Marian went with him, and they had a very pleasant week end. There was a large audience for his lecture at the Hopkins — "Goodness knows I was a little frightened when I saw all those dignitaries in the front row." (The dignitaries included Dr. Warfield T. Longcope, who had been Chief of Medicine at Johns Hopkins Hospital since 1921.) "They seemed to be pleased with my talk," George said, "and they were very kind to me afterwards. Baltimore is a remarkable place, and the atmosphere down there is always very pleasant, and particularly when it happens that you, the visitor, seem to know a little more about the subject than those who are listening."

He had had his eyes and ears open in Baltimore. The spring of the year is the time when all the professors are looking for good men to work in their laboratories, and when the young graduates are looking for good positions. He liked the looks of two young men who were about to finish their internships at the Hopkins and was pleased when Dr. Longcope spoke well of both of them. He was more pleased when both agreed to come to the Thorndike in September. His complement for the next academic year was filled—and ahead of time.

The Kober Medal, voted at the meeting at which he could not be present, was awarded to Dr. Minot at the meeting of the Association of American Physicians in May 1929. Dr. George M. Kober himself escorted George to a chair on the platform, and while George sat there quite ill at ease he made a very complimentary speech which included these two sentences: "His brilliant work in pernicious anemia was not a matter of chance or good luck, but must be attributed to his scholarly researches in diseases of the blood . . . Our congratulations go out to you, [Dr. Minot, with] the sincere hope that your years of usefulness to humanity may still be many and that it may be given to you and your coworkers to add fresh laurels to your fair renown."

When George stood up to receive the medal, he was well aware that some five hundred pairs of eyes were upon him. "I appreciate very much this honor . . . [and] I thank you," he began, and then went on, in part:

> Many individuals have given us assistance in the work. The delightful coöperation of Doctors James H. Means, Wyman Richardson, Henry Christian, William B. Castle at the different hospitals in Boston has enabled us to study many cases and thus permitted the work to progress relatively rapidly. Thirteen clinics in this country, one in Canada, and one in England assisted in testing out liver extracts so that a reliable preparation could be made available for public use. We and the profession are greatly indebted to them for their careful work.
>
> There is only one essential factor in the successful treatment of pernicious anemia, namely, that the physician be sure that the patient receives a potent preparation and obtains indefinitely enough each week. Satisfactory results depend upon optimal doses being maintained at all times . . .

George was pleased with Dr. Castle's work:

> An epoch-making discovery concerning human gastric physiology and pernicious anemia has been made by Dr. Castle. His study of about 22 cases suggests that normal gastric juice can unlock something from beefsteak necessary for the Patient with pernicious anemia . . .
>
> In conclusion I ask you to note that I consider this honor conferred upon me reflects upon many persons who have helped and taught me in

various ways, especially the late Dr. J. Homer Wright and Dr. Roger I. Lee, and my former chiefs, Drs. Edsall, Thayer and Howell; men who have taught me how science provides the means by which human suffering may be alleviated and who have aided me to understand fundamental knowledge and clinical problems.[10]

Activities at the Thorndike were increasing. Everybody was busy and happy, and the new experiments were working out well. The study of diseases of the blood was being advanced rapidly. "Our stock is going up!" was the way George put it.

Dr. Chester S. Keefer came to the Thorndike in 1930. A Hopkins graduate, he had been a resident at the Billings Hospital in Chicago, and then had spent two years in China as Associate Professor of Medicine at the Peking Union Medical College. He had always been interested in anemia: in the factors that cause it, like deficiencies in the intake of vitamins, minerals, and total food, or like the intestinal disorders — the dysenteries — found in the Far East, which interfere with the absorption of food elements. He was interested in the effects of anemia on the heart, on the peripheral nerves, and on the stomach. Needless to say, he was an important addition to the Thorndike team.

When Dr. Janet Vaughan, of Oxford, wrote George to ask if she might come to America to work in his laboratory and learn about his scientific advances, George was delighted to welcome her. He knew her by name, and had read some of her early papers. She was not only an attractive English lady but a good doctor who had become much interested in blood morphology.

Dr. Vaughan had been particularly impressed with George's demonstration of the reticulocyte response as a measure of bone-marrow activity. She could see how the response had provided a useful tool by which to measure Dr. Cohn's fraction of liver. After she came to the Thorndike, she began to talk with Dr. Gulli Lindh Muller, as well as with George, to see if the tool could not be perfected still further. What was needed was some method to test Dr. Cohn's fraction which did not require that tests be made on patients. The upshot was that they found that if common pigeons were raised on a diet limited to cereal grain, their bone marrow became quite inactive, and when they were injected with certain of the liver fractions, they gave good retioculocyte responses. At the time, the analogy between the response of apparently healthy pigeons and the response of human beings seemed a little farfetched, and the method was not further explored. In patients the reticulocyte method was good, and its general validity was soon demonstrated in another study.

Scurvy is a rare disease in this modern day, but it is found occasionally in elderly men and women, especially those who have lost their wives or husbands, who live alone, poor and discouraged, and whose diet contains very little vitamin C. The lack of vitamin C may cause anemia as a part of the general debility. Dr. Mettier found [11] that fruit, green vegetables, and fresh liver — foods that are rich in vitamin C — can cause in such patients a prompt response of reticulocytes and rapid regeneration of blood. Neither large doses of iron nor the substance potent in pernicious anemia appear to accomplish these effects. The bone-marrow factory needs raw materials of several kinds.

What Dr. William B. Castle called the "ubiquitous reticulocyte response" played its part in the third series of experiments carried on in 1931 and 1932. Dr. Clark W. Heath, the excellent student who was soon to go to Germany and England, was interested in "secondary" anemia, so called because it is the result of some other process. (It is also called "hypochromic" anemia, because the cells look pale under the microscope, and "microcytic" anemia, because the cells are of small size.) Chronic blood loss, as from small bleedings in the gastrointestinal tract, can produce a secondary anemia, and the special variety that stems from a lack of iron in the diet has been called "chlorosis."

Drs. Minot and Heath[12] showed that after the administration of iron, recovery was associated with a reticulocyte response quite as in primary pernicious anemia. The bone marrow could work quite well as soon as it was given iron to work with.

One night, George met Dr. George C. Shattuck at dinner, and by the fire afterward the talk was led around to the problems of anemia. Dr. Shattuck had written a paper on the similarities of beriberi, a fairly common disease in the tropics, characterized by weakness, prostration, and severe pains in the muscles, and the polyneuritis that develops sometimes in our New England climate. In both conditions the pains in arms and legs may be severe, and weakness of the muscles may be crippling. In both cases, the patients have lived on diets that are far from good. Dr. Shattuck suggested that both diseases might come from nothing more than poor nutrition, perhaps from the lack of a particular factor in the diet. George saw the point of this at once. The talk reminded him that his great-grandfather, Dr. James Jackson, had written a paper "On a Peculiar Disease Resulting from the Use of Ardent Spirits." [13] Dr. Jackson had thought that the symptoms of "neuritis" were due to a "poisoning" of the nerves by alcohol, producing an "alcoholic neuritis of toxic origin." Now Dr. Shattuck was pointing to a similar complex of symptoms, but this time due apparently to a deficiency of diet, and George Minot was delighted.

It so happened that Dr. Maurice B. Strauss and Dr. W. J. McDonald [14] had just completed a report on three women whose neuritis during pregnancy was proved to be not "toxic" at all, but the result of improper diet. When the women were made to eat properly, their pains disappeared. This result fitted into the discussion by the fireside. Here, then, was the beginning of another advance made by George's group at the Thorndike.

In 1933, Minot, Strauss, and Cobb[15] (Dr. Stanley Cobb was at that time Chief of the Neurological Unit at the Boston City Hospital) showed that all their fifty-seven patients with "alcoholic neuritis" had histories of defective diet and of chronic digestive disturbances; and that when forty out of the fifty-seven were treated with a diet rich in proteins, minerals, and vitamins, all forty were relieved of their pains. They concluded that "dietary deficiency, especially of vitamin B_1, plays an important role in the production of [the so-called] 'alcoholic polyneuritis.' " A few years later, Dr. Strauss[16] proved the effects of diet by showing that the disease stemmed from the lack of food and not the excess of alcohol, since the polyneuritis cleared up when the consumption of food was adequate, even though at the same time the patient continued his customary daily intake of spirituous liquor.

Disturbance of blood coagulation, which resulted in abnormal bleeding, had always interested George. Hemophilia is a blood disease of dramatic interest, for any break in the skin or mucous membrane of its victims may continue to bleed indefinitely, and after any serious wound the patient may bleed to death. The blood does not clot. Hemophilia is inherited, but in a peculiar pattern, in that only the female transmits the disease, while only the male shows its manifestation. It appeared in the royal families of Europe. Queen Victoria had five daughters and four sons. Three of her five daughters were carriers of hemophilia, and for the second daughter, Alice, the disease had important political repercussions. Alice, who married Prince Louis of Hesse-Darmstadt, had seven children, one of whom, Alexandra, married Nicholas II of Russia. When their son, Alexis the Czarevitch, developed hemophilia, the monk Gregory Rasputin claimed knowledge of a cure. The Czarina was gullible, like ordinary mortals, and she believed in Rasputin. With his smooth talk, the quack hypnotized her, and his influence came to extend far beyond his medical functions. Corruption in high circles was fostered by Rasputin until finally he was shot by Prince Youssopoff in 1916. The Czarevitch died shortly after that.

George Minot was always intrigued with this story. As he pointed out, it is interesting that none of Queen Victoria's four sons had the disease — at least Mr. E. F. Benson, writing about *Queen Victoria's Daughters*[17] says nothing about it.

In this modern day, thanks to the early research work at the Thorndike and later to the achievement of Dr. Edwin J. Cohn in separating the various fractions of the protein in the blood plasma, the defect in hemophilia has been found to be in the plasma, the fluid portion of the blood. More than that, Rosenthal[18] has recently reviewed the modern findings that the deficiency in hemophilia may be of any one of several factors in the blood plasma. One can almost consider it as a series of different diseases with different treatments for each one.

The Boston Daily Globe for September 24, 1954 has a story about the patient named Russell White, age forty-five, who had hemophilia. "He was brought to the Thorndike in 1932 by Dr. Minot and has been there ever since." The reporter, Mrs. Frances Burns, quotes the man: "When I came here, I was at a low ebb. Today I am perfectly well. Tomorrow I may feel a muscle sore and tight and a joint aching, and I know I'm bleeding into the joints again."

White's blood, studied so extensively, is used again and again to test the plasma of patients who bleed from unknown causes. If a small amount of plasma (say 0.10 cc.) from the specimen will clot 2.00 cc. of White's blood, then the patient has "antihemophilic activity" and is normal. If, however, no clot forms, then the patient may have hemophilia. During World War II, both the army and the navy sent samples of blood to be tested at the Thorndike, and White's blood was almost an essential tool. Russell White was much interested in this work. He was more than coöperative; he was delighted to play such an important role. Mrs. Burns quotes him again:

"Dr. Minot wanted to have someone always in the ward that could be used for his blood experiments. That's why I've stayed here . . . I remember Dr. Minot warmly. He was a kind man. He'd sit beside a patient and listen to him, let him tell him how he was feeling. He was soft-spoken. Like all the research workers, he'd usually end up by referring back to knowledge he'd got from reading, right back to the Bible."

Back in 1916 George, with Dr. Roger I. Lee,[19] had studied the platelets in hemophilia, believing that the trouble was a disturbance in their function. They knew that the transfusion of normal blood into a patient with hemophilia would restore the coagulation time to normal and stop the bleeding, for at least a day or two, and they thought that the result depended upon the normal platelets which had been injected. Twenty years passed before Patek and Stetson,[20] working in Minot's laboratory, examined the subject again in 1936 and showed that transfusion supplied platelets and other blood cells, to be sure, but that its real effect was to supply something in the plasma which could replace what they thought was a defective prothrombin. In 1937 and 1938 Dr. Patek and Dr. F. H. Laskey Taylor[21] found that the "something" was a globulin substance which was present in normal blood, but lacking in hemophiliac blood. Dr. Taylor, the chemist, showed that this globulin substance had nothing to do with either prothrombin or fibrinogen. After George retired, one of the many things that he liked to recall was the finding that in hemophilia the platelets are normal.

Purpura is another hemorrhagic disease that was studied under Dr. Minot in the Thorndike Memorial Laboratory. He wrote the section on purpura for Cecil's *Text-Book of Medicine*[22] in all its first seven editions. Purpura is a disease in which blood escapes from the vessels to make purplish spots under the skin. The spots are usually about the size of pinheads, but there may be "black and blue" areas 3 or 4 inches in diameter. Blood may extravasate into the tissue of the intestines or the kidneys, and it may be found in the stool or urine. When the bleeding is into joint cavities, severe pain — a kind of arthritis — develops and it is called "Schonlein's purpura," and when the bleeding is into the intestines it becomes "Henoch's purpura."

As George wrote: "The cases most difficult to diagnose are those in which visceral symptoms develop without skin lesions. The crises of pain [from hemorrhage into one or another internal organ] so closely resemble those of an acute abdominal emergency that operation cannot always be forestalled." [23] One can believe that George, who was quite aware of this possibility, successfully made the difficult diagnosis more than once.

There are several ways in which purpura is produced. In purpura simplex there is no trouble with the platelets or with the blood; the bleeding comes from leakage from capillaries, the walls of which have been injured by the toxic effects of fevers, drugs, or poisons. Purpura hemorrhagica, also called thrombocytopenic purpura (and this is a much more descriptive name since a thrombocyte is a platelet and penic means poor or few), is a very different disease. Here the platelets are at fault, and the whole mechanism of blood coagulation is impeded. The blood escapes spontaneously — that is to say, without obvious cause — from mucous membranes in the eye, the nose, the mouth, or the bowel. Again hemorrhages (purpuric spots) appear under the skin, and hemorrhages may develop in the internal organs. In this disease, the platelets are diminished in number, sometimes because a poison or toxin has injured the large cells in the bone marrow that make them, and sometimes by an antibodylike substance that develops in the blood plasma and can destroy them. Harrington[24] has recently demonstrated the validity of this theory when he injected into himself a small quantity of the serum of one of his patients. When he did this, his own platelet count dropped to zero, and he developed hemorrhages. Fortunately, they were not serious. One of George's assistant residents found several pregnant patients who had purpura and whose newborn infants also had purpura for a few weeks, a sequence that suggests that something — an antibody, presumably — passed through the placenta from mother to child.

Thrombocytopenic purpura, and purpura simplex also, may develop in severe fevers, in certain types of anemia or leukemia, as also in chronic poisonings as from benzol or arsenic, and an interesting group of cases stems from allergic reactions to drugs, or, rarely, to foods. The treatment of purpura of all kinds is easy in theory — "Find the cause and remove it" — but it is not always easy in practice.

These details about purpura are included here because they illustrate again how careful observation of a group of patients, with studies that compare one case with another, can lead to a classification of causes and effects, and so to the understanding of the process by which the disease is produced.

This account of the progress in science, of the discoveries in the Thorndike Laboratory, extends somewhat ahead of the story of Dr. George Minot, but then a good many activities were going on at the same time; George's life was complex, to say the least.

At the Boston City Hospital, the wards, both medical and surgical, are divided into Services, two for each of the three Boston medical schools — Tufts, Boston University, and Harvard — and each Service has two wards, a male ward and a female ward. The appointment of interns, residents, and visiting physicians and surgeons to each Service is given to the corresponding medical school, with the provision that all appointments must be approved by the trustees of the Hospital. In every city institution paid for by tax money, patronage casts its shadow at times, and George was troubled when he found that the men he wanted on the Harvard Services were not as pleasing to the hospital trustees as were some other men who happened to be better known to them. There were times when the difficulties flared to considerable proportions. It was Dr. Soma Weiss, or sometimes Dr. Locke, who would help to smooth over the controversy and end by having the best man appointed.

George worked hard on the proposition that the Second and Fourth Services, as well as 50 percent of the Medical Out-Patient Department, should be integrated with the Thorndike Memorial Laboratory, to make a complete Harvard Unit. Appointments of doctors to this Unit should be made by the Harvard Staff of the Boston City Hospital, who would also recommend the same men for teaching positions in the Harvard Medical School.

That he talked well, and that he was able to drive his point home, is shown by the end result: the trustees agreed to appoint him as Physician in Chief to the Second and Fourth Medical Services, in addition to his appointment as Director of the Thorndike Memorial Laboratory. Also, they appointed Dr. Locke as Chief of the Fourth Medical Service. Dr. William H. Robey was already Chief of the Second Service. George was delighted.

Other difficulties were not quite so vital. "The morale of the house officers is not all that it should be," George said. "The records are not up to date. The residents and students do not come on time for their visits. Either I am fussy and finicky, or else they are getting more sloppy in their ways — it is time for us to do something about it." Again it was Dr. Weiss who could talk to the young men, to help them rearrange the mass of routine work, to show them how to write their histories with fewer words, and to make them meet the Chief on time.

A little later George wrote to Locke about another matter: "What about that message, received the other day by the senior house officer, which directed that a certain patient is to stay another week? — Who runs your service anyway? — Who tells you, or me, whether this or that patient will go home tomorrow or stay another month? — What do they know about his physical condition? I do not like this interference at all."

Another time, he appeared on the Fourth Service unannounced: "Not a single patient on Ward U has been weighed. I have always felt very strongly that every patient, except those desperately ill, should be weighed on admission. The neglect, I think, is shocking. I was told that the proctoscope had not yet arrived, and that numerous articles, still on requisition, and needed badly, had not been received."

Another letter to Locke adds:

> I learned that notices regarding precautions, which used to be attached to the patient's bed, have been removed, for the reason that visitors do not like to see their loved ones marked in this special way. I was shocked, of course, and now I would insist that the order for special

precautions be posted at the bedside wherever they are needed. The whole problem of cross infection is much too serious to be neglected. I learned the other day that one of our patients with pernicious anemia, who happened to be in the next bed to another patient with a septic sore throat, acquired a sore throat by direct contact, and in her weakened condition the infection rapidly advanced until it killed her. The danger is very real. [Patients with] acute upper respiratory infections should be quarantined, and all special precautions should be taken to protect not only the other patients, but the nurses and doctors as well. The "preventive medicine" around here is rotten. I realize that the crowding in wards T and U makes isolation difficult, but still there is a good deal that can be done by screening and by the insistence on following the directions for precautions. The careless management sets a very poor example for the students.

This problem of the spread of acute infections in the hospital ward from one patient to another, and from patients to the personnel, was not easy to solve: "The Fourth Service has outrageous crowding. The wards in the new medical building were designed for 28 patients, and now they contain 40 patients. The side rooms, designed for four patients, have five extra cots in them. It is dreadful, but we are on record as protesting vehemently." His protest was heeded. Mayor James M. Curley was very sympathetic with the difficult problems of the City Hospital, and the improvements came after a time.

The frequent messages from City Hall, that such and such a patient is to be moved from a cot to a bed, were troublesome, and George tried to be patient in spite of his irritations: "We need only think of our own family in a similar predicament to feel sympathy for the relatives, but don't forget that our job is to take care of all of our patients as best we can, and City Hall must realize that we have to give the beds to those patients who need them most," he said.

There was a rumor in the Hospital that research work on the Second and Fourth — the Harvard — Medical Services had not been as great, either in quantity or quality, under Dr. Minot as it had been under Dr. Peabody. George didn't like that rumor, for it was so completely false. "Less research?" he said. "Look at the figures and you will find that the number of papers directly concerning patients coming from the Thorndike and the Fourth Medical Service in the past *two* years is three times the number in the *five* years before that time. Furthermore, the number of patients who have been studied carefully on the Fourth Service has trebled in the past two years."

Another rumor had it that Harvard was grabbing all the Boston City Hospital.

"That is not so either," Dr. Minot said. "Look at the figures. Harvard has increased its teaching force over here by 25 percent, but Tufts has increased hers by 473 percent. Back in 1909, about a third of the Harvard teaching was done at the Boston City Hospital, but now, in 1931, only 16.7 percent is done here. No! Harvard is not grabbing."

When Dr. William H. Robey and Dr. Franklin W. White retired from the Second Service, Dr. Minot emphasized that it would be quite desirable for the students to be brought in contact with these senior men, and he asked Dr. Weiss what he thought about arranging to have Dr. Robey and Dr. White continue to meet the students once a week through the winter. "The students," he said, "should enjoy the privilege of their experience and their wisdom."

Money for his laboratory was always short, and he looked for grants from various sources. Most of the money for research in the Thorndike came in large measure from the City Hospital itself, thanks to the logical persuasions of Dr. Francis Peabody at the beginning, but some of the work was supported by the Harvard Medical School, and occasionally extra grants for some special purpose were obtained.

In May George, reporting to Dr. Joslin about his diabetes, added a scrawl to his letter: "Mr. Lilly has given us a grant of $5,000 a year for three years for me to use. Isn't that wonderful? I hired a new technician this morning!"

"New money" like this advanced the work greatly. George had asked for this particular gift and was immensely pleased when it arrived.

An industrial company of New York offered a grant on condition that Dr. Minot and his group would work out certain problems that were important to the company. In reply George wrote an interesting letter:

> We are not in a position to have the . . . Company direct the studies or stipulate what should be done. Of course, we would consider your

desires and be pleased to talk with you from time to time. The . . . Company could not, of course, have any control over publication of results, nor could they be given permission to utilize unpublished information. You should realize that you would be in no way responsible for the results — it was not you who directed the studies — but by giving money to Harvard, the Company probably would find that useful information was obtained.

10

Extracurricular Busyness

In 1928 and 1929, business was good in America. Herbert Hoover was President, everybody seemed to have money, and everybody was employed profitably. Improvements in the automobile and in the roadways made it easier to move around, and to live outside the city became more practical. Many of George's friends were building homes on those sections of large estates in Brookline, in the suburbs of Boston, which had been sold for real-estate development. George and Marian, together with the Henry Minots, had been looking at an attractive property near The Country Club in Brookline, and finally they bought it.

The area was big enough for two houses with grounds and gardens, and the architect, Mr. John Radford Abbot, was commissioned to draw plans according to the general idea that George and Marian discussed with him.

In June 1929 the house at 30 Marlborough Street, where they had lived since 1922, was sold, and the family moved into 188, to stay there for the winter. This made an interruption — to put it mildly — for Cousin Jim; for it was not easy to take two busy people, with their two small children and the children's nurse, into the house to live with him. However, everyone seemed to survive.

The summer of 1929 was a hectic one for the Minots. The move to 188, and the plans for the new house, made extra interests and activities on top of a schedule that was already busy.

When the architect had drawn the first plans for the new house, it became apparent that time and attention must be devoted to them if the finished house was to be satisfactory. George did not mean to be fussy or different from Mr. Abbot's other clients, but the fact is that he *was* different, and the business of trying to please him in every little way was not too easy. The plans had to be redrawn not once but several times. The details were important: "In that closet under the stairs, we should have shelves for rubbers and overshoes, and in this corner — isn't there room for another little closet with more shelves for tools and light bulbs and such things? Where shall I keep liquor? Wouldn't that be a good place? If so, tell Abbot to make the shelves high enough for bottles underneath." (The house was to be permanent. Prohibition was to be temporary — he hoped.) "In our dressing room upstairs I want a small sink and an electric outlet for my sterilizer. Should the outlet be on the right side or the left side? Should those glass doors go all the way across or be divided?"

"Hours with the architect bring matters so that the contracts can be opened for bid sometime in August — we expect," George said to me.

In July the whole family went to Northeast Harbor once more, to the same house under the fir trees. In early August my wife and I went up to join them, and we had a wonderful six days. They had hired a Friendship sloop, with Captain Harvey, a typical State-of-Mainer, to sail it for them, and almost each day we would go off on an expedition, with our lunch and fishlines. George always enjoyed these little cruises. We would sail out through the "Western Way," and anchor in the lee of a lovely little island, and then we would go ashore to explore the place and go in swimming — all except George. He seemed to be in good condition, but one day he had a fit of weakness and trembling, which was quite distressing. It showed once more that when his blood sugar became too low, he could be in real trouble.

In late August 1929, the International Physiological Congress was held at Harvard. Distinguished scientists came from almost every country in the world to attend a program that lasted for a whole week. That was the time when the famous Russian physiologist, Professor Ivan Pavlov, a great friend of Dr. Walter B. Cannon, had traveled alone through New York and in the Grand Central Station this "absent-minded professor" had had his pocket picked. Here he was, this distinguished scientist, eighty years old, Nobel Prize winner, the man who had discovered the important principle of conditioned reflexes (the first demonstration of the effect of emotion on bodily function), all alone amid crowds of people in the enormous building, wanting to take the train to Boston but now with no ticket and no money. Fortunately, he had the wisdom to telephone to the Rockefeller Institute, and they in turn had the good sense to send a young assistant with a roll of dollar bills: "Run to the Grand Central Station as fast as you can and find Professor Pavlov." The old gentleman had to wait over one train, but he arrived in Boston, where Dr. Cannon met him at the station, his body safe in American transportation but his mind confused by crime, generosity, and hospitality coming in much too rapid succession.

The program of the Congress listed short papers which were classified according to their subject matter into sections, and meetings of the sections were held on each of the five mornings in the week. More formal lectures and addresses were presented in the afternoons to the Congress as a whole, and in the evenings, except Tuesday, there were entertainments, including a special concert by the Boston Symphony Orchestra.

George did not himself address the Congress, but his friend Dr. Edwin J. Cohn presented a report of progress on "The Nature of the Material Effective in Pernicious Anemia," [1] in which he gave full credit to Dr. Minot and his associates for their essential help in evaluating the chemical fractions as they were produced and purified in Dr. Cohn's laboratory.

The program allowed for one free evening. On Tuesday Drs. Minot, Means, Weiss, and Rackemann gave a dinner at the Brookline Country Club, each inviting six of the visiting delegates. The four of us had a pleasant luncheon ahead of time when we chose the names of twenty-four foreign members more or less at random, except that there were to be not over two delegates from any one foreign country. The result was exciting, and we had a most interesting evening. I remember sitting with the Director of Public Health in Finland on one side and a professor from South Africa on the other side. I do not recall George's neighbors. Dr. Means was toastmaster, and his first problem concerned language. Should he talk in English, French, or German? To settle it, he asked for a show of hands and learned that everyone could understand English except the two gentlemen from — where do you think? — France! On the next night came the Symphony Concert, and although

George himself knew very little, and cared very little, about music, nevertheless he described it as "an extraordinary occasion — a truly beautiful affair — totally unique." On Friday he had fifteen clinicians come to see him in the Thorndike Memorial Laboratory, "and never in three hours did I learn so much." There was, however, one discordant note, for one of the visitors — "a peculiar looking man," George said — seemed to have the idea that the bone marrow was not the place where blood was made; it was the place where the old worn out blood cells were removed from the circulation. It took a few minutes of valuable time to prove to him why he was so wrong. The others were quite amused.

On Monday, August 26, George and Marian went back to Northeast Harbor, to stay until a week after Labor Day. On the back of a letter he wrote: "I have rented one of the new Fords, a truly splendid machine." (It was a "Model A.")

At the end of the summer, the plans for the new house seemed to satisfy everybody, and on Monday, October 26, the contractors started work. On Sundays in the fall and winter of 1929–30 the family would often motor out to Brookline to survey the progress of construction. "I think it is going to be good," George would say. "The placing of the house is just right, the sun will come in all day, and do you see that big ash tree? It is far enough away so that its branches cannot keep out any light, don't you think? We want to keep these big maples on the north side to break the wind, and the workmen have been good about protecting them."

"You will plant trees to shut out Henry's house?" I inquired.

"Yes! — Henry's house does look pretty close, but with several evergreens of good size in the space between, I doubt if we will know it is there."

By March 1930, the new house was nearing completion rapidly, and the little girls were excited at the prospect of sleeping in their own rooms. George and Marian were excited too. All the time and trouble spent on fussing over little details was very trying for the architect, but it paid off, as one might expect, for when the house was built, it was found to be ideal. The living room was of good size, with a fireplace at the end. It was on the sunny side, with windows looking out at what would someday be a garden. The dining room was next to it. The kitchen and pantry were modern and convenient. The doctor's library was most attractive, with bookcases extending from floor to ceiling on two sides. The dark woodwork and the fireplace made it a cozy place to enjoy good talk or quiet reading. The sunroom, with benches for plants, had doors opening into it from both parlor and library.

Charles Sedgwick Minot, George and Marian's son, was born on March 18, 1930. He had come a little ahead of schedule, and he was allowed to stay on at the hospital for several weeks after his mother had gone home. He gained rapidly and was very well.

In May the painters were putting on the finishing touches, and finally all was ready. On Monday, May 26, the George R. Minot family moved in, and young Master Charles Sedgwick Minot came too — straight from the hospital on a lovely, warm, and sunny spring morning.

Furniture from storage, furniture from 188, trunks, bags, babies' bassinets, nurses and servants, with their own trunks and bags, all arrived together, and the movers tracked in dust and dirt with every load. It was quite an experience, but friends gathered round and worked hard so that by nightfall some order had been produced and supper could be prepared and eaten. Marian and George were satisfied that a good job had been done well. They were delighted to find that the house, which they had tried so hard to make perfect, really was almost perfect. It was a happy day. Even the baby seemed to like it.

The grounds around the house were developed later. Marian Minot knew about plants and flowers almost as much as George did, and together they arranged the two gardens. The one by the house had handsome perennials selected to make a show of pretty flowers, beginning with the tulips in early spring and ending with the asters and chrysanthemums in the fall. Down beyond the big ash tree was a picking garden, with a large bed of roses and another of annuals. Several good-sized Scotch pines and yews were set out, and on the north side of the house the laurel and rhododendrons came to look as though they had been there always. Christmas roses — those lovely white flowers which continue to grow regardless of the weather — were appealing, for in the early winter the first frost and snow did not hurt them; there they were blooming away, even under the white cover.

When he lived in the city, George had liked to browse in the back alleyways, just as he liked to browse in the book stores, and particularly in and after the Easter season. "Look what I found today — three pots of perfectly good bulbs sitting on top of an ash can in the alley just back of this house. The flowers and leaves have dried up, of course, but don't the people realize that they can keep the bulbs until next fall and then make them flower once more? To be sure, they won't be quite so good as the new bulbs straight from Holland, but they will do for planting out of doors."

Around the new house, under the trees and beyond the lawn edge, they planted daffodils of all kinds — jonquils and narcissus in variety, with occasional hyacinths mixed in. (They did not all come from the city alleyway!) Some years later these bulb plants had spread to make a lovely show in the early spring.

Dr. A. B. Meikeljohn, a British visitor before the war, remarked on the beauties of the American flowering dogwood trees that stand outside the Minot home, and expressed surprise that the tree was so seldom seen in England. Some months later, on returning to England, he was amazed to receive a consignment of three young dogwood trees — a present from George.

George's special hobby was his irises. Beginning about 1932, he started collecting different varieties. In his travels to medical meetings, he had found that Dr. Frederic Hanes at Duke University, Dr. Graves in Concord, New Hampshire, Dr. David P. Barr in St. Louis, and Dr. Russell M. Wilder at the Mayo Clinic were also interested in irises and were delighted to trade their duplicates so that each man could improve his collection. Each year the iris garden was more handsome than the last, but it took work to make it so. The rhizomes (roots) were divided with great care, and the new plants were set out and labeled carefully. A good many roots were given away, and many friends, myself included, have lovely irises in their gardens because of the generosity of George and Marian Minot.

George learned the technique of cross fertilization. With a fine camel's-hair brush he would transfer the pollen from the anthers of one flower to the pistil of another and then cover the bloom so fertilized with a piece of light cheesecloth to keep out insects who might contaminate the artificial union. Then he would stand up, brush the dirt off his hands, look at his handiwork, and exclaim:

"There now! Don't pick or injure that flower on your life! With a little luck, we'll get a seed, and then we'll plant it later." Needless to say, this new seed was guarded and nursed with great care, and its planting was labeled with name and date. It took two years for the new plant to mature until it produced a flower, but then the interest and excitement of seeing what this new flower was going to look like more than compensated for the long "incubation period."

Each spring the show produced by the irises was handsome, it is not surprising that prizes for the "Best Iris" and for "Best Arrangement of Iris" were won at the Chestnut Hill Garden Club and at the New England Iris Society shows.

Whenever the expert talks about his own field, whether it is science, or horses, or irises, his enthusiasm makes the talk worth hearing. At one of the meetings of the Medical Exchange Club, George talked about irises. The yellow iris is the fleur-de-lis of France; the Japanese iris is the common blue flag. The German iris — the tall, bearded variety — is a cross between the wild iris of Italy and the wild iris of Hungary. Our common Easter lily is really a special form of white iris. It originated in the Mediterranean, and not in Bermuda as so many believe. When the roots of wild iris are dried and powdered, the resulting orris root is used in cosmetics, chiefly because of its soft texture and its pleasant smell, George explained, but the Secretary added that since certain individuals develop an allergic sensitiveness to it, the better preparations do not contain orris any more.

For some years George had been quite friendly with President Lowell of Harvard. Mr. Lowell knew all about his family, and he had always been pleased with George — and all the more so since that Commencement Day in June 1928, when he had conferred the honorary degree upon him. It is not surprising that Mr. Lowell knew something about his illness, as well as about his struggles at the City Hospital.

In February 1931, George wrote to Dr. Joslin:

> Mr. A. L. Lowell is troubled about me — the Dean has similar thoughts, and gossip has it that they wish to do something that will prevent me from having such a load of administrative work and duties

that do try the soul. To be in charge of 21 full-time men, 13 half-time men, 200 beds, etc., is a load. I have, of course, not actually seen a case at the hospital since December 1, owing to illness and administrative duties.

Just what the authorities have in mind, I will tell you when I know. I will see Dr. Edsall tomorrow.

Needless to say, the authorities told him to carry on but to try to slow down a little and not take on extra activities. The advice was timely, because his ambitions were likely to outrun his strength.

It was easy to show that fatigue played an important part in all his symptoms, and it was quite remarkable to observe the change in all parts of him when summer came and he could be in Maine.

In August 1932, he wrote me from Northeast Harbor:

I await the evening insulin before dinner . . . The afternoon you left us, Marian and I trotted up to the waterfall at the base of Sargents. On the way back a deer leaped forth, crossed the path and rushed on through the thick young white pine. On Tuesday, we sailed on Rodman Peabody's schooner over to the Schoodic Islands and back — a perfect day — and on Wednesday we sailed in the morning and went to the sand beach in the P.M., where Charlie [aged 2] had a grand time. Today I caught eight flounders, 2 codfish, and 4 perch off the harbor buoy in a row boat.

When George was back at work, the pains in the legs began again, so that in September 1932 Dr. Joslin sent him for consultation to the surgeon, Dr. Leland S. McKittrick. Some atrophy of the left calf was found; the left foot was distinctly colder than the right, and there was a definite level — about two inches above the ankle — where the temperature seemed to change. Dr. McKittrick suspected that he had a thrombosis of his left popliteal artery, which was causing what is known as intermittent claudication. A little later his bad feet were to get him into real trouble.

When Dr. Henry A. Christian realized in December 1932 that the Hersey Professorship of the Theory and Practice of Physic at Harvard was about to have its one hundred fiftieth anniversary, he realized also that each of the six former incumbents had a direct descendant who was now on the staff, and so he arranged a commemorative meeting.

The occasion was academic,[2] and Dr. Christian conducted it with great solemnity; he made the speakers wear caps and gowns. To George fell the honor of presenting the account of his great grandfather, Dr. James Jackson, who served as the second Hersey Professor from 1812 to 1836. He began by reading this text of a vote:

> That the Faculty [of the Harvard Medical School] recognize with gratitude the labours of Dr. Jackson in removing the medical school to Boston, in obtaining a building for its accommodation, in his lectures in Theory and Practice and on clinical medicine, and in effecting the establishment of the Massachuetts General Hospital and connecting it with the Medical School . . .

And then George went on:

> Jackson was considered a conspicuous and popular teacher but not a brilliant one. He taught the practical as well as the scientific side of medicine. "His patient was the man and not the disease."
>
> He wrote as he taught, saying the most useful things in the simplest way. His "Letters to a young Physician" [3] (1855) are full of practical guidance for the student today . . . He prescribed cod-liver oil with whiskey, but since these two ingredients do not remain well mixed, he commonly found the whiskey gone and the cod-liver oil in the bottom of the glass!

At Christmastime 1932, George wrote me a formal letter, on formal stationery this time:

> I'm sorry that I could not get in [to your house] this P.M. but my leg has been annoying me more lately. I wanted to thank you for your gifts . . . especially since in one I read that for legs like mine a bit of rum with regularity is of positive value. Being at home alone, I am having visions. I have visions of studying more intensively the social aspects of medicine with a view to . . . teach medical social service to students. I have a desire to write on "The Care of the Patient" from the point of view of the need for precise directions. To tell the patient to eat food is not enough: one must tell him exactly what food, how much, and when. And then I want to write up the history of Lobelia, discovered first by Rev. Dr. Cutler of Ipswich . . . and I ought to be busy writing up some back work on familial thrombosis, iron absorption, arsenic in P.A., the treatment of nervous disorders complicating P.A., etc., but the extraneous topics seem at the moment more interesting — the plants, the butterflies, and medical history. How can one in one lifetime do all that he would like to do?

Whenever George had a good student that he liked, he was always interested in him and was ready to help and advise, even at long range. In 1933 Dr. Clark W. Heath went to Europe to study under Professor Marowitz at the University of Leipzig, and he sent back several good letters which pleased George. In the spring of 1933 Hitler was gaining power rapidly, and Dr. Heath reported that the freedom of thought and speech, which had made the work in German clinics and laboratories almost as productive as work at the Thorndike, was being curtailed. The atmosphere was changing, and he wrote to Dr. Minot: "I do not want to have you disappointed in me, but if you could see the conditions here, I believe that you would agree that I could spend my time much more effectively if I went to England."

George replied: "It is hard for us here to know the circumstances. Please feel free to get out of Leipzig, and when you arrive in London, go to see Dr. Donald Hunter and Dr. Janet Vaughan."

A few days later Heath heard from Dr. Hunter: "I have heard from Dr. Minot that you are thinking of leaving Leipzig prematurely. Nothing would delight us in the London Hospital more [than to see you] . . . Don't forget that if you come, there are many besides myself who are anxious to pick your brains."

Here at home the men at the Thorndike were doing excellent work. Dr. Richard B. Capps came in 1933. During his two years' residency, he learned about research and laid the foundation for his work on acute disease of the liver (hepatitis) which made him an authority later on.

Dr. Maxwell Finland, who came to the Thorndike in 1928, has worked there ever since, pursuing his studies of the infectious diseases and the bacteria that cause them. He is a quiet fellow with a keen sense of humor which keeps the atmosphere normal. Meantime, he is an authority on the mechanisms by which penicillin and other antibiotic drugs produce their dramatic effects.

Dr. Wesley W. Spink and Dr. Thomas Hale Ham were appointed in 1934. Dr. Spink has told me more than once of how much he learned and profited by his three years under Dr. Minot. He is now Professor of Medicine at the University of Minnesota. It is fair to say that he knows more about brucellosis, sometimes called "relapsing fever," than anyone else in the world. Dr. Ham was, and is, a very able and active investigator, with a brilliant mind. He worked more directly than the others with both Dr. Castle and Dr. Minot on the blood diseases. Today he is Professor of Medicine at Western Reserve University in Cleveland, where he and Dr. Wearn have undertaken a radical experiment in medical education. The basic principles and facts of man's structure, his functions, growth, and behavior, and his relation to his surroundings, are studied together and then correlated and unified by instructors who point to the differences in people and the different ways in which they react to the disease process. With the new point of view, the results of chemical and physiological measurements become more interesting and more understandable.

George liked to go to medical meetings. He liked to meet again his many friends who lived in other cities. He wanted to know at first hand what those who had worked at the Thorndike were doing in their new positions, and then he wanted information about new young graduates who might be interested in coming to the Thorndike. Equally important, he wanted to learn of those academic positions which might be open to those who had finished their residency under his guidance. Personal conversations on the Board Walk in Atlantic City, where the Association of American Physicians meets each year in May, often lead to the fitting together of man and position which works to the great advantage of both.

These conversations often began on the train going to the meeting. Dr. William S. Middleton's letter to me recalls a typical incident:

Dr. Minot could become so absorbed . . . as to forget time and occasion. We were engaged in earnest conversation on one trip from Philadelphia and were just coming to the salt flats outside of Atlantic City when Dr. Minot jumped up with the exclamation, "By George, I forgot I had my wife aboard. I shall have to run back and find her!" Just another example of the absent-minded professor.

On frequent occasions I have referred to Dr. Minot as an intellectual grasshopper. You will appreciate that there was only high admiration and no thought of demeaning his intellectual capacity and habit. Yet times without number, I can recall discussing clinical and hematologic problems with him, areas in which I should have had superior grasp, only to find him leaping hither and yon into discussion of details that should have occurred to me without his prompting. Ours was a very happy association, but I fear one in which the advantages were largely unilateral. I am ever grateful for the friendship of this great American physician.

There was one medical society which was quite different from "The Association" and which appealed particularly to George. It had an interesting origin. In 1874 Dr. Edward L. Trudeau, seriously ill with pulmonary tuberculosis, established himself in a little red cottage at Saranac Lake, New York, and he did not die; he slowly recovered most of his health, so that he could found the Sanitarium which accomplished so much and achieved such fame. He and others became convinced that climate was important in medicine. In 1884 they founded the American Climatological Association, and it prospered. Forty years later, in 1924, Dr. Gordon Wilson of Philadelphia, the new president of the "Climatological," emphasized that sound training in general medicine was essential for all specialists. By opening its programs to other topics besides diseases of the lungs, he changed the character of the Association. The word "Clinical" was placed before "Climatological" in the name. For many years, the Association was managed largely by its Secretaries — Dr. Guy Hinsdale from 1895 to 1918 and Dr. Arthur K. Stone from 1918 to 1933.

George Minot joined the "Climatological" in 1925. In 1933 he was elected President, and in that same year Dr. Stone resigned his Secretaryship. George had the authority to appoint a new Secretary, and he appointed me. Dr. Stone was pleased with this arrangement, and said to us: "The 'Climatological' is a remarkable group of friends. They are all good fellows and they will do whatever you tell them to do." To me, George said: "Here is a wonderful opportunity. Let us see how this Association can be improved still more. First, we must continue to choose new candidates with greatest care. Let us try to find scholars who have culture and charm, and then let us find attractive men who are scholars." We discussed a second important matter and agreed that the President, rather than the Secretary, should be responsible for the program — for the number, the selection, and the arrangement of formal papers. In that way each President can set the tone of his own meeting. Many amendments to the Constitution were made, and at the next annual meeting all of them were voted without question.

Emphasis on the two principles has been important ever since, and the "Climatological" has become an important influence in American medicine. Its membership includes most of the important professors of medicine in this country, and the papers read at its meetings are of high quality.

In his Presidential Address in 1933, George talked on "The Importance of Art and the General Principles of Treatment in Chronic Arthritis." [4] "The physician must take infinite pains to delve deep into the patient's life . . . [He] must make free use of the imagination [as does] the poet or artist . . . It is the play of the imagination that permits rearrangements so necessary for the chronic invalid." And then follows an exhortation to prescribe rest, exercise, and especially food in their proper forms and quantities. The sentence at the end is good: "To teach the art of courageous living is often the chief prescription for the patient with chronic arthritis."

In 1936 the American Clinical and Climatological Association set up the Gordon Wilson Lectureship, partly to recall the name and the character of Dr. Gordon Wilson and his contributions to the Association, and partly to encourage some distinguished investigator to come each year and talk at some length about his field of interest. Several times the lecturer has been one of the members. The first lecture was given by Dr. Warfield T. Longcope in 1937, and the second by Dr. Henry A. Christian in 1938. The third lecture was given by George R. Minot in 1939, when he presented the discussion of the "Anemias of Nutritional Deficiency," [5] and that remains as a classic paper.

When the new laboratories of Eli Lilly and Company in Indianapolis were to be dedicated in October 1934, George was invited to join the company of distinguished guest-speakers, which included Sir Frederick Banting, Dr. George H. Whipple, Dr. Elliott P. Joslin, Dr. Irving Langmuir, Dr. Carl Voegtlin, Dr. George H. A. Clowes, and Sir Henry H. Dale.

George's address[6] dealing with the clinical investigative laboratory included these phrases:

> Wards with patients are the salient feature. It is from . . . [the records of consecutive data] that concepts regarding the nature, the treatment, and the prevention of disease are formulated . . . There are two types [of clinical investigators]. The first is the trained clinician who

seeks his tools to solve his problems which originate at the bedside; the second is the trained technician who takes his tools to the bedside to solve, let us say, chemical problems. Both types . . . have their place . . . [but if only technicians are present], the practical needs of clinical medicine are apt to be forgotten.

Clinical ability and scientific curiosity are essential, George said, adding that the clinician may need help from many sources.

I need only cite the excellent example of the splendid coöperation of Eli Lilly and Company with the Harvard Committee on Pernicious Anemia . . .

Investigative work has a large educational value. An understanding of the principles of investigative work can lead [the physician] to judge critically, to appreciate the . . . significance of . . . controls, and to distinguish the chaff from the wheat.

His favorite line was included:

The diagnosis of the person is too often neglected when diagnosis of the case is made in detail . . . The science dealing with the relation between human behavior and health is in its infancy, and the progressive physician should attempt to advance medical knowledge in that direction . . . For the clinical investigative laboratory, man in all his manifold relations will remain the center of thought and action.

In Indianapolis, the Minots stayed with Mr. and Mrs. Josiah K. Lilly, and the Lillys remember the visit well. Not only were the Minots very good company and very appreciative guests, but "they were so observing and so inquisitive," said Mrs. Lilly to me. Mr. and Mrs. Lilly live in a beautiful house on the outskirts of the city. Back of the house is a garden, and beyond it the lawn slopes down to a creek. One of Dr. Minot's first questions was: "What creek is that? It connects, I suppose, with the White River which runs into the Wabash — Mrs. Minot and I have been studying the map."

Mrs. Lilly had to confess that she was not too sure about the creek, but she found an early map, drawn when Indianapolis was just beginning to develop, and she and Dr. Minot learned that the creek back of her house was once a canal that led up to a limestone quarry. George was pleased to have had a part in finding this new information. Mr. and Mrs. Lilly were delighted.

Between 1931 and 1936 there was correspondence with Mr. H. B. Logie of New York concerning a new nomenclature of diseases. A national conference had been arranged, under the guidance of Dr. Haven Emerson of New York. If the nomenclature of disease, which implies accurate definitions, could be standardized and adopted by every hospital, studies of a particular disease made in one place would be comparable with those made in another place. In theory the idea was good, but to make it work was another matter.

Almost every specialist could find some fault with the nomenclature in his field, and it is not surprising that George was disturbed about the classification of the anemias. "The term 'aplastic anemia' has caused confusion," he wrote. "Some, like myself, consider that it means an anatomical aplasia in the complete sense, while others use the term to indicate a functional physiologic aplasia in which the marrow can make the cells well enough but for some reason cannot deliver them into the circulation." As he pointed out, new knowledge changes the definitions frequently, and this is the trouble with nomenclatures.

Another matter that is sometimes annoying to busy people is the recurrent request for biographical data: "We are compiling a new Encyclopedia — please be good enough to fill out the questionnaire enclosed," a letter would say. On one occasion, Dr. Minot wrote: "My biographical sketch has been published in a considerable number of encyclopedias of one sort or another. I thus am referring you to *Who's Who* [and] *American Men of Science* . . . You will also find data concerning me in the reports of the Harvard Class of 1908 on file in the Widener Library."

George hated publicity. When one day in 1930 Paul de Kruif asked for an appointment to interview him about the story of The Discovery, which he proposed to include in his book *Men Against Death*,[7] George was not at all pleased. He soon appreciated, however, that the story was going to be written anyway, and so he gave time to Mr. de Kruif and was as polite and considerate as possible under the circumstances. The resulting account was exaggerated in places, but not badly exaggerated.

Worse yet was the later time when the Pathé News came to take pictures of George at work. "Goodness knows what a lot of contraptions they brought along," he told us at dinner that night. "Why, my office looked like a machine shop before they got through. And down in the ward they upset the routine scandalously. They had me examining a patient, and that was all right until I turned back the bed clothes, not too carefully, and found that the man had an umbilical hernia as big as a balloon. We couldn't possibly show that to the public — could we?"

"What did you do?" I asked.

"I covered him up as quickly as I could, but I guess it was too late. However, the Pathé man assured me that he would take out all frames that might be objectionable. Goodness knows, there was some excitement on that day!"

In the nineteen-thirties, George's achievements were being recognized more and more. In 1930 he received the gold medal of the National Institute of Social Sciences, and in the next year he and Dr. W. P. Murphy learned that they had been awarded the Cameron Prize by the University of Edinburgh and were expected to go over to Scotland in May 1931. A little later Dr. Minot and Dr. George Whipple were awarded the prize of the *Popular Science Monthly,* amounting to $5,000.

In 1933 he was awarded, by the City of Philadelphia, the John Scott Medal, which bears on its face the words, "To the most deserving," and in the same year he received the Moxon Medal from England.

When Dr. Walter Moxon of London died in 1886, a fund of money was subscribed and given to the Royal College of Physicians in trust. Every third year the Moxon Trust awards a medal "to the person who is deemed to have most distinguished himself by observation and research in Clinical Medicine." As the prospectus says: "The award, which is not restricted to British subjects, is made by the College on recommendation of the Council . . . and the Medal is presented to the recipient on the occasion of the Harveian Oration."

The Moxon Medal itself is a handsome gold piece, which George Minot treasured for the signal honor to him which it represented. He was the fifteenth recipient and the first American Moxon Medalist.

George said very little to his friends — even to me — about these new evidences of the recognition that his discovery had engendered, but when we happened to see the announcement in the newspaper, and then asked him about it, his satisfaction and pleasure were obvious.

11

Nobel Prize

It was late on Wednesday afternoon, October 24, 1934, and on the third floor of the Thorndike it was quiet. Almost everybody had gone home. George was still at his desk in his office in the corner room, and Dr. Richard B. Capps was in his laboratory down the corridor. The two were alone when the telephone rang.

George picked up the receiver with his usual reluctance, disturbed once again by the interruption.

"Is Dr. Minot there?"

"Yes, this is Dr. Minot."

"This is the American Scandinavian Society in New York and I have a message for you from Stockholm, Sweden. Please stand by for a conversation that will begin in about ten minutes." Nothing was said about the nature of the message.

"What could Sweden want?" George asked himself. "Dr. Nylin? Dr. Holmgren? Yes, I have corresponded with them. Perhaps some important person is sick and the doctors want expert opinion." He was thinking fast, and he dashed to the corridor and called to Dick Capps:

"Oh, Dick, come in here quick and help me."

George's thought was that Dick could find papers with data and figures if necessary, but Dick had visions of a heart attack, or perhaps a hemorrhage, and he came running.

"I think that someone in Sweden is trying to talk to me on the telephone," George said. "I haven't the slightest idea what they might want, but I wish that you would stand by me until I hear."

Dick Capps was much relieved to find that George had not had a heart attack and that the trouble was only his customary anxiety about an imminent, perhaps difficult, situation for which there was no time to collect his thoughts. The two men sat wondering what might be going to happen next. After a few minutes the telephone rang again. There was a good deal of clicking, but presently a voice said:

"Is this Dr. Minot? This is Mr. ——" and George never did catch the name "in Stockholm, Sweden. I am very pleased to tell you that you have been awarded the Nobel Prize in Physiology and Medicine for 1934. Dr. William P. Murphy and Dr. George H. Whipple are to share it with you. We want to have an interview with you; just a minute, please."

After more clicking another voice came in and said, "This is London." And presently other voices said, "This is Paris," "This is Berlin," "This is Rome." And then a more distant, feeble voice said, "This is Tokyo," and an "awfully jolly fellow" said, "This is Sydney, Australia." Then, finally, ordinary American voices said, "This is San Francisco," and "This is New York." At that point, the first reporter explained that a world-wide hook-up with reporters in all the capitals of the world had been arranged, and now he would like to ask Dr. Minot a few questions.

By that time George's heart was pounding, his face was flushed, his eyes were flashing, and he was trembling slightly. Dick was excited also, and he moved over to put his head near the receiver, so that he could listen in.

"How did you happen to discover the liver treatment, and when?"

The question was easy, but to be called upon suddenly and without the slightest warning to phrase the answer in a few well-chosen words over a tremendous world-wide hook-up, within a space of about five minutes, was not so easy. However, the voice was very reasonable, and George rose to the occasion beautifully. When the next question concerned the latest number of patients and the latest reports about the liver fractions, Dick was able to find the papers without too much trouble. So soon as he could turn to the right page, the latest figures were plain to see.

When the conversation ended, all George said was, "Well, I'll be damned!" He really was overcome, and it took a little while for the full meaning to sink in. Slowly, he collected his thoughts.

"Stay here a minute until I call Marian, and then we'll see what to do next," he said to Dick.

When Marian came on the line, he said: "Marian! Listen to this! And listen carefully! I have just had a long-distance telephone call from Sweden. Someone told me that I, with George Whipple and Bill Murphy, had won the Nobel Prize. What do you know about that?"

"What did you say?" Marian found it hard to believe what he had told her.

"I say that Whipple, Murphy, and I have won the Nobel Prize!"

"What do you mean? Nobel Prize, did you say? I can't believe it!" Marian began to be excited, too. "Who told you about this? Who did you talk to? Do you think it's really true?"

"Yes, I guess so!" George said. "I'm coming home right now. Sharkey [the chauffeur] ought to be here and I'll tell you all about it. Don't do anything or say anything until I get there."

George had not been at home very long before the telephone began to ring.

"Is Dr. Minot there?"

"Yes," Marian answered. "Who wants him? Is it important?" And then she said to George, "One of those newspaper men wants to see you in your office."

She said into the telephone, "Dr. Minot does not go to the Hospital in the evening."

Then she listened for a moment, and said to George, "He says it is quite important. There are a number of reporters, and they all want to ask you about pernicious anemia so that they can write their stories — what shall I tell him?"

"I imagine that they will print something anyway," George said, "and we had better see that what they say is at least somewhere near the truth — but I don't like the idea very much; we were looking forward to a quiet evening. But — all right, tell them to come out."

The interview was much less of a trial than either he or Marian expected. They were pleased to find that the reporters seemed to know something about pernicious anemia and about liver, and that they were kindly, considerate fellows. It was not at all hard to talk to them; in fact, George was pleased with their interest and with their intelligent questions. It was not the flattery that impressed him; it was the satisfaction of finding outsiders who seemed to appreciate so much what had been going on in the hospital and laboratory under his supervision.

Next morning both the *Boston Herald* and the *Boston Globe* had headlines on the front page: "Dr. Minot to Share in Nobel Prize with Dr. William P. Murphy and Dr. George H. Whipple." The *Herald* had a picture that showed Drs. Minot and Whipple, dressed in their best, receiving the *Popular Science* Annual Award back in 1930. The *Globe* had a picture of George at his desk in the Hospital. Each paper had a dramatic story, which began: "Dr. Minot received the news while he was standing at the bedside of a sick patient. Only nine days ago this man was dying but 'by means of a needle we injected liver extract into his system and tonight he is sitting up, shouting for food.'" That afternoon the *Boston Evening Transcript* had a similar account.

On Friday, October 26, a formal radiogram was delivered to George at the Medical School. It was dated Stockholm, October 26, and it read:

THE CAROLINE INSTITUTE HAS DECIDED TO AWARD THIS YEAR NOBEL-PRIZE FOR PHYSIOLOGY AND MEDICINE TO PROFESSOR G MINOT DOCTOR W MURPHY AND PROFESSOR G WHIPPLE JOINTLY FOR THEIR DISCOVERIES CONCERNING LIVER THERAPY AGAINST ANAEMIAS

GUNNAR HOLMGREN RECTOR OF THE CAROLINE INSTITUTE

The accounts in the Sunday papers were all that George dared to hope for. He could see that this newspaper publicity was not an advertisement; it was a sincere effort to tell the public about the work, and he began to believe what the reporter told him: that when a discovery as basic and fundamental as this is made, the public has a good right to know about it, and that it is for the best interests of the investigator to tell the whole story, and tell it correctly. He is quoted this way:

> Others thought that in pernicious anemia blood was destroyed too fast. I chose to think that blood stopped growing. Patients would get better for a while and then there would be a relapse which progressed. Always the result was fatal — in about three years. It seemed to me, for various reasons, that the victims needed something special in their food, and I thought about the liver, which Dr. Whipple had been giving to his dogs. I started treating patients, and Dr. Murphy joined me in 1925.

A year later we found that most of the 45 cases treated with liver were doing well. Instead of dying, — they lived; but they had to eat about eight ounces of liver a day, and that is half a pound, and it is a big amount to ask a patient to eat. And so the next question was to find the nature of the substance in the liver which was producing the result. Dr. Cohn evolved an extract of liver of which a tablespoonful was as good as the eight ounces of whole liver. Still later this crude extract was purified further until it could be injected by needle into the muscle, and in this form it was thirty times as effective as the first crude extract given by mouth.[1]

The statement was simple, and it was easy to understand.

Winners of the Nobel Prize are expected to go to Sweden to receive it. George's first reaction to the idea of such a trip was doubt about the wisdom and safety of a man with his disease traveling so far, and in winter. "You and Dorothy will go with us, won't you?" he asked me. "Just think of the fun that the four of us could have together." Then he added, "You would be there to help in case of an emergency."

The invitation was tempting, but a few days later I had to tell George and Marian that we could not go with them. Fortunately, however, it was soon found that Dr. and Mrs. Richard P. Stetson would be delighted to accompany the Minots. Dr. Stetson had been one of the brilliant young men under George's tutelage; he and his wife were delightful people.

Dr. Joslin told George that he must get a permit to carry insulin with him, so that the customs officers would not be so curious as to unpack the sterile containers.

Letters and radiograms of welcome, anticipating George's visit, began to come from England, Holland, France, and other places. Most of them wanted Dr. Minot to stop over to give a lecture, so that doctors and students could see and hear the great man. Yes, he was going to Sweden, there was no doubt about that "—and we had better get busy," George said. They booked passage on the *New York* (Hamburg-American Line), which was to sail out of New York at midnight on Wednesday, November 14. Time was short, and to say that the Minot family put in a busy three weeks is, at best, an understatement.

Finally all was ready, and George and Marian, with their daughters — Marian, then sixteen, and Elizabeth, thirteen — accompanied by Dick and Dorothy Stetson, left Boston on the train at noon on November fourteenth. Charles, aged four, was left at home. Between them, the party had seventeen pieces of luggage, including the old slouch bag with the scales, the syringes, the insulin, and several blocks of blue paper. The Minots had never been able to travel light! In New York, they had a gay dinner at the St. Regis Hotel. George bought a bottle of sherry to take with him, but when the taxi was being unloaded at the pier, the sherry dropped to the pavement. The bottle broke, and the whole party broke into gales of laughter, much to the amusement of the bystanders. A porter said that it was good luck, but George was not so sure, and he had lost a perfectly good bottle.

Their staterooms on the *New York* were very comfortable. In one, there was an enormous pile of packages: flowers, fruit, books, and bottles in variety — sherry included — presents, and tender messages from friends. Three newspaper reporters appeared, and bothered George with questions and flash pictures. He thought that they would never go ashore and leave him alone.

He was quoted as saying: " 'Tell debutantes and stenographers that they should eat more of the proper foods. Pastry and chocolate milk shakes,' he snorted, 'that's a fool diet! . . . Many young women would be astonished to learn how run-down they are because of a deficiency in diet resulting largely from the desire to keep a trim figure. We want young women to eat plenty of meat, milk, fruits, and leafy vegetables.' "

On the sixth day at sea, George wrote me a letter:

> How you would enjoy this trip! It all seems like a dream. It takes me back 26 years [to that other trip with classmates in college] . . . I have completed my outlines for the lecture to the staff of Guy's Hospital on November 27, my paper for the Royal Society of Medicine on November 29, and then the Nobel Lecture, which comes on December 10. Also, I have tried to write a good speech for the dinner in Stockholm.
>
> Yesterday we visited the bridge. I watched for an hour beside the wheel, absolutely fascinated, and today the Commodore let me steer for about ten minutes, with him watching like a cat beside me. There were two officers on the other side and a sailor behind. We were yawing plenty and it took 3 or 4 turns of the wheel to straighten her out again. The compass has a magnifier which shows one-hundredths of a degree. . . .

The man who prints the ship's newspaper got orders by wireless to take my picture for the German papers.

On Thursday, November 22, the party landed at Southampton. Dr. Janet Vaughan came out in the tender to meet them on the ship, and, thanks to her, they passed through the customs without delay. George was pleased to see how easy it was to let the porters move the party from ship to train, and all the bags were accounted for. At the Park Lane Hotel they found many invitations awaiting their arrival.

Four days later, George wrote me again:

To think of me ten years ago [and then to know] that I am here in London as gay as a lark is remarkable. Went to Cambridge on Sunday by motor to lunch with the Regius Professor of Medicine, Dr. W. Langdon Brown . . . On the way back we stopped at Saffron-Walden, where the Minot family first began; saw two Mynott graves, dated 1754 and 1806, near the church.

Marian's scrapbook continues the story: "In the afternoon Dr. Brown showed us Queen's College, King's College, and Caius until quite suddenly George developed a 'reaction,' and was forced to retire to the motor car, which, fortunately, was not far away. With a couple of crackers and a lump of sugar, he was 'better.'" Even in England, he had to be very careful of his food — to eat neither too much nor too little. Incidentally, Marian had great trouble with his syringes. The hard water made the insulin precipitate; bottled water became necessary. What a nuisance is diabetes!

George's letter goes on: "Tomorrow I lunch at the London Hospital and speak at Guy's [Hospital]." The scrapbook contains a broadside announcing his lecture, and Marian's note says, "The audience was large and very appreciative."

We have appointments for all of the days before we leave for the continent at 2 P.M. on November 30 [George continued]. I have been obliged to refuse fascinating invitations, including one to the Anniversary Dinner of the Royal Society, of which Sir Henry Dale is President . . . On Tuesday is a luncheon with Sir Arthur Hurst, to see his clinic. On Wednesday I meet Dr. [Sir] Francis Fraser at Bart's [St. Bartholomew's Hospital], and that evening I discuss some of the papers of the Royal Society of Medicine.

. . . And so it goes. How we wish you could be with us. It is 11:45 P.M. and I must get to bed, as it has been after 12 for five days before our lights were out. We have invitations galore in Amsterdam and Copenhagen, and I wonder if we can do it all.

On Friday, November 30, the Minots left London. As they were trying to leave the hotel, a doctor wanted to see George about his patient, a member of the Royal Family with pernicious anemia. George had no time to give him except in the cab on the way to the station. Life was extra hectic. As usual, he was worried about the train schedules, about the tickets, and, above all, about the luggage.

The arrival in Calais was uneventful, and France looked good. At the Belgian frontier, they had to pay duty on the bottle of alcohol that George used for wiping his arm before the insulin injection. They did not reach Brussels until 8:30 P.M. The girls were tired, and poor George was exhausted! Next day, they went on to Amsterdam, where Professor Isidore Snapper, leading authority on blood disease, met them at the station.

On Sunday after lunch, Dr. Snapper took George and Dr. Stetson to his hospital, where George had a very profitable afternoon, and the interns enjoyed their distinguished visitor and what he said about the little details of diet. On a postcard, George reported, "A wonderful time with Snapper yesterday — extraordinary show at his hospital."

That night all six "Minots" dined with Dr. and Mrs. Snapper in the Snappers' apartment, Mrs. Snapper having discussed with Marian the need for food of any particular kind. Most of Monday and all of Tuesday were spent on the train, with a "quick sleep" Monday night in Hamburg. "A great effort to get the children and George up — to catch the 8:52 A.M. train for Copenhagen," Marian said. The long day was broken by two crossings between the Danish islands, with the whole train on the ferry boats. The thick fog was disappointing, for George couldn't see where he was going.

At Copenhagen, the Minots were relieved to find Dr. and Mrs. Einar Meulengracht on the platform. They are charming people. They had been in America, so that to see them again was to meet old friends. Photographers met them also, much to George's annoyance, and other reporters were waiting at the hotel.

On Wednesday, December 5, it was raining, but Dr. Meulengracht came in the midmorning to take George and Dr. Stetson to his Bispebjerg Hospital. George asked questions about everything, and learned much. In the afternoon, he lectured to the staff and students at the Rigshospitalet across the city. In between times, he spent an hour in the Thorwaldsen Museum, where he observed that the first lion that the sculptor made had a cow's tail; the second, however, had a normal lion's tail. How did he know about that? How keen and how inquisitive he was!

That evening, they all dined with Dr. and Mrs. Meulengracht and were delighted to meet a number of important doctors. "We all had a good time but got to bed late," Marian notes. And George's pencil adds, "very very much too late!"

Dr. August Krogh, the distinguished physiologist who had been in Boston at the Physiological Congress in 1929 and who had taught several of our friends, had written to George in London, inviting him to visit his laboratory, to stay to lunch, and then to dine at his home in the evening. George had a most interesting day with Professor Krogh. At the dinner that evening, he met Professor Hagedorn, who was in charge of one of the units producing insulin in Denmark.

On Friday, December 7, the Minot cavalcade left Copenhagen, crossing the Sound to Malmö, where an electric train took them to Stockholm. After a long eight-hour journey, Professor H. C. Jacobaeus ("tall, dark, and handsome," Marian says), Chairman of the Medical Nobel Committee, met them at the station. The ubiquitous reporters were there, too, saying, "Tell us all about yourself" — in five minutes! A grand suite, complete with sitting room, had been reserved at the Grand Hotel, and several bouquets of flowers, with cards attached, stood on the table there.

George had had a letter from Mr. Laurence G. Steinhardt, "Envoy Extraordinary and Minister Plenipotentiary of the United States to Sweden," which said: "There are certain customs and formalities [concerned with the Nobel Ceremony] and I thought it might be advisable for you and Dr. Murphy and Dr. Whipple . . . to have a talk with me."

Dr. and Mrs. George H. Whipple had sailed over on the *Albert Ballin,* and the Minots were delighted to find them in the same hotel. Dr. and Mrs. Murphy were there also, so that on Saturday afternoon they could all go together to the tea at the Steinhardts' for a talk around the table. George was pleased to learn even more about Alfred Nobel and his prizes.

Alfred Nobel was a scientist; he was not a financier. As a chemist, he discovered nitroglycerine and its properties — and the discovery brought him both fame and fortune. Before his death in 1896, at the age of 63, he conceived the idea of his prizes and willed that the income from his fortune should be spent for them. Curiously, however, he did not specify how the money should be cared for and distributed, and so it happened that the King of Sweden appointed a Nobel Foundation and retained the power of making new appointments to vacancies on its Board. There are five Nobel Prizes — in physics, in chemistry, in physiology and medicine, in literature, and for the propagation of peace. The Peace Prize is awarded in Norway, but has not been given regularly. The prize in physiology and medicine is awarded by the Caroline Institute, one of the four Swedish medical schools. The professorial staff of the Institute, headed in that year by the Professor of Medicine, Professor Israel Holmgren, determine the recipient of this prize, and in doing so they pay great attention to the advices and comments which they invite from all previous Nobel laureates, as well as from many important doctors and scientists from all over the world.

On arrival in Stockholm, each of the new laureates was given a Memorandum of Instructions for the Ceremony on Monday, December 10, and Marian has told me that the program was carried out precisely as outlined. The Memorandum begins:

> The Nobel laureates, with their families . . . will be escorted to the palace from their hotel [the Grand Hotel] by an attendant, Count N. Tolstoy. Owing to the possible congestion of traffic round the Concert Hall, it may be advisable to start from the hotel at 4:30 P.M. Autos will be reserved for the purpose and will be in waiting before the Grand Hotel at the fixed hour.

The Minots, the Whipples, and the Murphys took plenty of time to dress — the ladies in their loveliest gowns, the gentlemen in white ties, white waistcoats, and tails. When Count Tolstoy came to help them into the Royal limousine, their excitement increased. The girls, Marian and Elizabeth, and also Dr. and Mrs. Stetson, went with George and Marian in the first car; Dr. and Mrs. Whipple and Dr. and Mrs. Murphy followed.

At the Concert Hall they were shown into a special room, where the three doctors waited for King Gustav V. Marian, with the girls and the Stetsons, was shown into reserved seats in the orchestra section just behind the Royal Family. The Memorandum goes on:

> At 5 P.M. sharp His Majesty the King, with the members of the Royal Family accompanying him, is expected to leave the parlour reserved for them in the Concert Hall and enter the large assembly hall. Their arrival will be announced by trumpet calls, thereafter they are to be greeted by the royal hymn.

When the King and the members of the Royal Family had occupied their seats, then the laureates entered the hall through the center doors in the back of the platform (the stage), "their arrival being likewise announced by trumpet calls." George was conducted by Professor Holmgren, Dr. Murphy by Professor Jacobaeus, and Dr. Whipple by Professor Gunnar Liljestrand, Secretary of the Nobel Committee; Mr. Luigi Pirandello, the Italian playwright, recipient of the prize in literature, was conducted by Dr. Hallstrom, Secretary of the Swedish Academy. It was unfortunate that Dr. Harold C. Urey, Professor of Chemistry at Columbia University, New York, could not be present. He had been awarded the Nobel Prize in chemistry for his discovery of an isotope of hydrogen that he called "deuterium," which, combined with oxygen, made "heavy water." The prize for physics was not awarded in 1934.

After making their reverence to the King, the laureates took seats in the front row of the right-hand side of the platform, looking toward the audiences; their conductors sat immediately behind them, and the Nobel Prize laureates from previous years who happened to be in Sweden were behind that.

Marian has several excellent photographs in her scrapbook. George is sitting very erect in the front seat by the central aisle. Next to him is Dr. Murphy and then Dr. Whipple, with Mr. Pirandello on the end. The stage has four levels, to make each row of chairs behind a little higher than the chairs in front. Marian has told of the deep-red carpets and deep-red velvet draperies, against which the white shirts and waistcoats and the white flowers at the sides stood out to make an impressive scene. On each side of the center aisle there were about twenty distinguished men and a few women, the laureates on the right, the Foundation members and distinguished guests on the left. Another photograph shows the audience — every man in his white tie and tails, every lady in evening dress with jewels plentiful.

The King sits in the front row center, and it is interesting to hear that the only time when the King ever stands up for anyone else is when the entire company stands as the laureates enter the hall.

The Memorandum continues:

After the salutary oration by the President of the Board of the Nobel Foundation, the proclamation of the laureates will take place in speeches held by:

Professor Palmaer for the receiver of the prize for Chemistry;

Professor I. Holmgren for the receivers of the prize for Physiology and Medicine;

Dr. Hallstrom for the receiver of the prize for Literature.

At the end of every speech in Swedish, followed by a short address in the language of the respective laureates, the laureate in question will be asked to step down from the platform in order to receive from the hands of His Majesty the King the Nobel gold medal, the diploma, and an assignation for the prize. The three laureates in Physiology and Medicine, Messrs. Minot, Murphy, and Whipple, having received jointly this year's Nobel prize in the said domain of science, will please step down together to receive, each of them his Nobel medal and diploma, and in common, the assignation for the prize.

Marian's diary adds:

When Professor Holmgren finished his proclamation of the three laureates in Physiology and Medicine, given in Swedish, he turned to them and spoke in English, and they walked across the platform and down a little flight of stairs. The King presented each, beginning with George, with a gold medal and a beautiful illuminated diploma in a leather binding, shaking hands a long while with each one and speaking a few words. When George moved away, he went up the steps sideways so as not to turn his back to the King and backed across the stage to his seat, turning his head at intervals to make sure he didn't hit something. Mrs. Meulengracht was kind enough to say that he was graceful.

The dignity and solemnity of the occasion must have been very impressive. What other government recognizes those individuals whose intelligence and — yes — inquisitiveness, combined with persistent endeavor, have contributed significantly to the welfare of mankind? How often does a King pay homage to the citizens of another land?

When George Minot returned to America and talked to us, we could see that he was still moved and stimulated by that one remarkable ceremony. He would never forget it.

But there was more to come. After the ceremony in the Concert Hall, the laureates and their families were conveyed to the banquet in the City Hall (Stadshuset), beginning at 7:30 P.M. The laureates, their families, the foreign ministers present, and some other persons occupying the places of honor at the main table in the banquet hall were asked to assemble in the "Prince's Gallery," entering through "The Hundred Members' Vault" on the left hand after passing the central court, where they were presented to H.R.H. Prince Gustav Adolph, the heir presumptive, and to the other members of the Royal Family.

The Stadshuset is the handsome building that appears in many pictures of Stockholm. It stands at the water's edge; the lower floor has an arcade around it and in the corner is a massive square brick tower with a graceful cupola at its top.

The great hall is called the Gold Hall, its walls being covered with gold mosaic. At one end is an enormous figure of a woman, the "Spirit of the Baltic," holding Stockholm in her hand. The head table along one side was set with 44 places, and ten long tables extended from it, providing seats for 348 persons altogether. The Minot daughters sat opposite each other at the central table, not far down from the head table. One may imagine the sensation of sitting at the head table in such a place and under such circumstances. The order of events at the banquet was announced in the same Memorandum.

When the dinner was well started, Governor Hammarskjold, the President of the Nobel Foundation, offered a toast to His Majesty the King in a few well-chosen words. After that H.R.H. Prince Gustav Adolph proposed a toast to the memory of Alfred Nobel, and the company rose to its feet again. Some minutes later on, during a pause in the banquet, Professor Liljestrand, Secretary of the Nobel Committee, made a speech on the significance of the prize as it applied to all the Nobel prize laureates in common.

The Memorandum requested that:

"The laureates, should they wish to return an answer to this speech, will please proceed in the following order, viz:

1. The laureate in Literature.
2. The laureates in Medicine or one of them, representing also the other two.
3. H.E. the Minister of the United States of America [Mr. Laurence Steinhardt].

All the speeches were announced to the assembly by trumpet calls. George wrote in pencil on the Memorandum that "We all spoke about 4 to 6 minutes each."

When his time came, George spoke as follows:

Your Royal Highnesses, Your Excellencies, Ladies and Gentlemen:

Medicine disregards international boundaries. The physician studies for the benefit of mankind. Alfred Nobel, by the expression of his lofty ideals, has recognized the importance of science and creative accomplishments in augmenting human happiness.

This honor which has been conferred upon the three of us is an honor to American medicine and to the men who created the scholarly environment in which we have found ourselves. The award illustrates the generous spirit of the Swedish people. In accepting this honor, I give recognition to those men who have taught me how science provides the means by which human suffering may be alleviated and who have aided me to understand fundamental knowledge and clinical problems: — such men as the late James Homer Wright, William Sydney Thayer, and Francis Weld Peabody, and also David Linn Edsall, William Henry Howell, Roger Irving Lee, and Edwin Allen Locke.

As each bit of information adds to the sum of human knowledge, it is evident that it is the little things that count; that give all the fertility and characer; and that give all the hope and happiness to human affairs. The concept of bigness is apt to be a delusion, and standardizing processes must not supplant creative impulses. In clinical investigation the sick individual is at the center of the picture. The physician must have a deep interest in his patient's economic and social structure as well as in his physical and psychic state. If attention is not paid to the diagnosis of the person the clinical investigator is apt to fail in studies of the patient's disease. Without a consideration of the patient as a human being, it would have been difficult to have fed patients daily large amounts of liver.

This honor serves as a great stimulus for me to continue trying to advance knowledge for the prevention and adequate treatment of disease. It also stimulates me to aid young men [to] become wise clinicians and investigators.

We in America are grateful to Sweden for the important role she has played in the progress of the scientific world. The intellectual spirit which pervades today's ceremonies insures the permanence of Sweden's progressive influence upon international art and science.[2]

On the day after the Ceremony, the Minots got up slowly and enjoyed a leisurely breakfast. They went sightseeing and were delighted with the little narrow streets and the quaint houses in the old part of Stockholm around the Royal Palace.

On that Tuesday evening they were to dine with the King. George observed that the handsome notices about this, sent separately to him and to Marian, were invitations, and not Royal commands. In the late afternoon George took some time to dress, for again it was important that he look his best, that he make a good impression. He and Marian rode over to the palace with the Whipples and Murphys in the royal limousine, the Stetsons and the girls not being invited. About eighty people were present, most of them men — distinguished professors, members of the Cabinet, as well as the gentlemen of the Royal Family. The long room was magnificent with its priceless tapestries and its cabinets filled with beautiful china and glass. The lackeys wore gorgeous livery covered with gold braid. An orchestra played during dinner from the balcony at one end. The King skoaled various people, including the Nobel laureates. Mrs. Minot was taken in to dinner by Prince Charles, brother of the King, who was head of the Swedish Red Cross and much interested in its problems. His wife was the Princess Ingeborg, sister of the King of Denmark, a very attractive lady, who was most gracious and kind to the Minots all through their stay in Stockholm.

After the dinner, all the guests went to the Soirée at the Musée National de Stockholm — "de 21 à 23 heures" (9 to 11 P.M.), where there was another reception. They found the girls and Dr. and Mrs. Stetson there before them. The Director of the Museum escorted them through the galleries, and at the end George and Marian signed their names in an elaborate guest book. George enjoyed the cordial, friendly contacts with important people quite as much as did his wife.

Wednesday, December 12 — the day of the Nobel Lecture at the Caroline Institute — George got up very late — only in time for a comfortable dressing and a "brunch" before going to the Institute. The buildings for the medical school and hospital were all new, modern in every way. They are on the top of a small hill, with a large view of the city. The scholarly presentation which George Minot made to the members of the Institute and their guests that day has been published under the title "The Development of Liver Therapy in Pernicious Anaemia: A Nobel Lecture."[3]

On Wednesday evening, the Minots and the Stetsons dined with Mr. and Mrs. Steinhardt, and had another very pleasant evening. Professor Holmgren was there, as well as the two distinguished chemists, Commander Arne Tiselius and Professor The Swedberg. On that same evening the Italian Ambassador gave a musicale. The Minots were pleased to go with the other laureates, but they were so exhausted by the many festivities that they had to retreat to the hotel as soon as the musical program was ended, foregoing the supper afterwards. Thursday was easy. There was a pleasant small luncheon party given by Professor Einar Keys, and the Minots enjoyed talking again with Professor and Mrs. Jacobaeus. The Murphys were there, also. After the party, the Minots packed, and sent flowers to many of their new friends who had been so kind to them.

George and Marian have given us vivid descriptions of the wonderful hospitality of the Swedes. Their dinners are formal. On arrival, each gentleman is given a card which requests him to escort a certain lady to her chair. "Skoals" are important. Each gentleman must skoal every other person at the table, holding up his glass until he catches his or her eye, and then continuing to look until, after a sip or two, his glass is back on the table. When dinner is over, the gentleman escorts his lady out of the dining room, and at the door they both shake hands with the host and hostess, and then shake hands with each other — a very pleasant ending to what is always a very pleasant and happy occasion.

The Minot party left Stockholm on the train at 11 P.M. on Thursday, December 13, the Whipples going with them. George was tired — he was exhausted — and so was Dr. Whipple. It was a dreadful night, the train was bumpy and rough, and worst of all, they were forced to get up at 7:30 A.M. so that the berths could be made up, although they were to be in the same compartments all the day. The four hours on the ferry provided a slight break. They arrived in Hamburg at 8 P.M., after dinner on the train, and then had to wait until 9:30 for another train to take them on to Bremen. It was midnight again before they were in bed.

The *Europa* sailed from Bremerhaven at 3:30 P.M. on Friday. The boat train left Bremen at 1:30; there was time in the morning to purchase a pair of Zeiss binoculars and a good camera. A North German Lloyd captain had heard that Dr. Minot was sailing on the *Europa,* and he came on board with a bunch of roses — his wife had been cured of her pernicious anemia by the liver diet. Both George and Marian were surprised and delighted by this kindly gesture.

What a pleasure to be going home and to have so many wonderful memories to take along! For the the next few days they could all relax. That night the entire party slept really well — for the first time since landing in England!

The passage to America was the roughest in some time. They passed through several storms, so severe that the giant ship had to lie to all one night and parts of two other nights. Speed was reduced greatly; one day they made only 242 miles instead of the usual 640 miles. Pictures taken by the ship's photographer next morning, when the storm was over, show the waves coming over the bow of the ship. It must have been quite a sight. After the first night, all the portholes were closed, and that was not too pleasant, but fortunately no one in the Minot party was seasick. Poor Dr. Whipple, however, was sick with an infection; he stayed in his bed all the way back.

One night at 10:30, when they were drinking beer in the smoking room, word came that the *Europa* was going to the rescue of a ship in distress. When they went out on deck, there she was — the *Sisto,* a Norwegian freighter, with her rudder broken, wallowing in the seas with her lifeboats all washed away. Four other liners had come to the scene. The *New York,* which happened to be one of the four, had arrived first, and she took charge. She had put oil on the water, and then she had launched a lifeboat, and after an exciting struggle, its crew succeeded in taking the sixteen men off the wreck. The other boats lay to, to windward, trying to break the force of the wind and the sea as much as possible. All the while, the *Europa's* powerful searchlights illuminated the scene. The ships stayed by for a while, but finally when there was nothing more to be done and the wreck had to be abandoned, the bigger ships moved off, leaving a tanker to stand by. To see the assemblage of these great vessels, and to realize how the wonders of radio had made the ocean small and friendly, was most impressive. George could understand and appreciate the unselfish, wholehearted coöperation, as well as the expert seamanship, that made the rescue possible. Another saga of the sea had ended.

On Sunday, December 23, the *Europa* docked in New York at 9 A.M. She was forty-eight hours late. Taking the train to Boston was an easy matter. Not even George worried about the transfer across the city or about the tickets on the Boston train or especially about his bags; but, by golly, all seventeen of them, including the little old slouch, were in a row on the platform when they stepped off at the Back Bay station in Boston.

12

The Professor — in Full Stride

When George returned from Sweden, his general condition was good; the stormy crossing on the *Europa* with two extra days at sea had provided a radical change of scene, needed badly by each member of the party. Dr. Stetson reported to Dr. Joslin that the trip had been a great success and that Dr. Minot's health had been good all through the difficult month; the diabetes was no problem.

A dinner was given in his honor by the Tavern Club, and Dr. Wearn has told me about it. President A. Lawrence Lowell of Harvard and President Karl T. Compton of Massachusetts Institute of Technology were both present, along with about fifty other distinguished leaders in business and education. Dr. L. J. Henderson was the principal speaker. He was pleased with George's recognition of Whipple's work and the part that Whipple's studies in his laboratory had played in George's own thinking, especially about the importance of liver as a source of nutriment for the bone marrow. The solution of problems in the clinic must depend upon advances made in the laboratory, as Dr. Henderson said, and the clinical investigator is wise when he can recognize the importance of those researches which may appear at first to be abstruse and irrelevant but which on further examination are found to have a fundamental bearing on the problem at the bedside. The old rivalry between the professors of physiology, chemistry, and pathology working in the laboratories in the Medical School and the professors of medicine and surgery working in the hospital wards and in their offices had subsided as soon as each group discovered how much it could learn from the other.

Back at the Thorndike, George was in good spirits. He was learning to take life easier — to let his assistants attend to more and more of the details for him. To realize that he had stood before kings, as the Proverb says, gave him a confidence that had not been quite certain before. He had had an experience that was unique among all his associates.

Each morning, his chauffeur drove him in town and landed him at the small back door in the basement of the Thorndike Building, so that he could sneak up to his office by the back elevator. He had almost a fear of meeting unexpected people "who might want to talk about some useless topic which would take my time." He rarely arrived before ten o'clock, for, as he often explained, "I am never any good in the morning. My system is such that I have to start the day very slowly, and you know that I never make appointments before ten o'clock."

His secretary, Miss Curtis, would open the large amount of mail before he came in, and he would look it over. Plans for the day were very important. "What time do I meet Dr. So-and-So? Is there a conference today? Do I go to the Medical School this afternoon or is that tomorrow? No! Tell this man that I cannot possibly see him now; I cannot see him until next Tuesday."

He did not like "surprises" — unexpected meetings or questions when he had not had a chance to think about them in advance. This, however, depended somewhat upon who it was that wanted to see him. If he liked the man as a person, and respected his work, he was always glad to talk with him, but if there was another who did not appeal to him quite so much, he would greet him for a moment and then ask Miss Curtis to arrange a better time. Always, however, he was polite, courteous, and dignified; he never offended anybody intentionally.

On many days his chauffeur would call for him at 12:30 and take him across town to 188 so that he could have "luncheon" — not just "lunch" — with his father, or to the Tavern Club, or perhaps to a luncheon meeting of a committee; but on other days he would take his meal alone in his office. The tray, with the food all weighed and measured to the prescribed amounts, would be brought up to him by the nurse-dietitian in the Thorndike ward on the floor just below his office. While eating alone, he would often take his shoes off and toast his feet in front of his electric sunbowl, for that gave him real comfort. He would have liked to invite someone to lunch with him tête-à-tête, but he was eating food specially prepared and served by the dietitian, and in that sense he was a patient rather than a patron. If a visitor did come in, he was given a chair and a cigarette and was encouraged to talk while the Chief ate — and listened. When George was alone with a young man, he might still take his shoes off. He might even stretch out on the sofa, and if the telephone should happen to ring, he would curse gently. He could always understand, could "read between the lines," and he had that rare gift — he could give his full, undivided attention to his visitor as he listened hard. If he did not like the person, there was no extra small talk, and the meeting ended promptly. If, however, a real friend came in, the talk was more likely to be about "the geese I heard last night," or about the laurel bushes in the hospital yard, or "Did you notice the colors in the center of each flower?" than about the problem that had brought the visitor in.

He was lucky to have Dr. Castle and Dr. Weiss to talk to about many problems. "Young Dr. X. does not seem to be getting on very well," George would say. "How can we help him? We have to persuade him that he is old enough not to need detailed guidance. He must learn to sail his own ship along the course that he himself has charted." Another time he asked, "I wish you would tell me what to do about the business of collecting masses of data about counts of blood cells and platelets and reticulocytes. I understand that Dr. Y. has been talking to Miss Daland, and wants her to help him with all his counts." (Miss Geneva Daland was — she still is — the senior research technician in hematology, and a very important member of the Thorndike team. She had worked with George at the Huntington and had moved to the Thorndike with him.) "We must tell him and tell her that there is too much routine around here as it is. This work should be done by the general laboratory of the B.C.H." and then, after looking out the window for a minute, he went on, "Let me say two things while I think of them. First, let us not measure any quantity of bloods in a purposeless manner. Let us have a clear-cut reason for doing it. Put it this way: instead of doing miscellaneous work and collecting miscellaneous data, let's get these new men to answer specific questions, and then make them take time to think about the results, to analyze them, and then to write a paper, and button it up. The other thing is Miss Daland again. Her most important duty is to teach house officers, residents, and graduates how to do blood work quickly, easily, and accurately. It was with that idea in mind that I was able to get her appointed here in 1928. To ask her a simple question is all right, of course, but if anybody expects to spend more than two hours with her, Dr. Castle or I should be informed, and we will decide whether that person is to be taught."

George was always writing notes. Whenever he had an idea — and that was "about once every hour or so" — he would write it on a slip of paper, any old paper — a piece of yellow block, or the edge of an advertisement torn from a magazine, or perhaps a postcard. It was not very often that he used a "good" piece of paper like a letterhead. The writing was often in pencil, and all too often it was only experienced people who could read it.

One note says: "In re your paper — you should add more discussion . . ." And another: "Did you see the paper by . . . ? What have you to say re the paper on reticulocytes in *Arch. Int. Med.* which refers to your work? I am puzzled. Please report about this at Staff Conference." And then a note to Dr. Castle says: "What about heredity and diabetes? — Why do 12 percent of P.A. patients have diabetes in close relatives?" He added: "This is written lying flat on my back on the sofa on Sunday." His mind was always two jumps ahead of his pencil.

When he had time, he would walk into one of the laboratories, and say cheerfully: "Good morning, Doctor, what are you doing? Goodness knows that looks complicated to me. No, don't try to explain it all; I might not understand it anyway."

"Those are thin slices of rat liver in that inner chamber, Dr. Minot, and we are measuring the chemical changes in the surrounding fluid to see how the enzymes in the liver produce their effect."

"Ah, yes. Now I know! That's the Warburg apparatus." George began to study the setup. "Let me see. This tube carries oxygen into the chamber, and what makes the whole business look so complicated is only the bottles and the tubing and the 'heater' required to keep the chamber at the proper temperature."

"That's right; it looks more complicated than it really is!"

On another occasion, he went in to see Dr. Heath and Miss Daland, and found them bemoaning the fact that a fresh blood smear had been left lying face up on the desk all night and the flies had eaten most of the blood. However, there was a little of the smear left, and they had stained it anyway. "Lo and behold," they soon saw that the flies had eaten the red blood cells but had carefully avoided all the white cells. George came in at precisely the moment when they were worrying about the loss of a valuable specimen. He did not care about that; on the contrary, he was delighted with this "accident," and he began to discuss the idea that here might be a clue to the old problem of how to separate the reds from the whites easily. Accidents have led to discoveries, but in this case the possible lead was not followed up.

George was always interested in the total over-all picture of each disease, and therefore he was fully aware of the importance of the out-patient department in a teaching hospital, for there the students learn what happens to ward patients after they leave the hospital.

For the young graduates in medicine, however, work in the general medical out-patient clinic has never been satisfactory. There is never enough time or opportunity to analyze any one case completely and, more important, the great variety of diseases and symptoms that must be treated interferes with the chance to study any one group of patients with similar problems. George appreciated this, and occasionally he would appear in the Out-Patient Department in the hope of stimulating the men to make their work more thorough, and therefore, more interesting to themselves. His coming would please the young men and the patients alike. One morning, a rather puzzling case demonstrated the importance of "being able to see what you are looking at," as he explained in no uncertain terms. The patient had a peculiar pigmentation of the skin. George bent his tall, thin frame to a right angle, squinted his eyes, and then wrinkled his nose and turned with a slight air of disgust: "Don't you know what that is? If you asked me, I'd say it was just plain dirt!"

His correspondence was enormous. There were letters from everywhere, sometimes accompanied by blood smears on glass slides, asking advice about patients. To each letter George replied with care, so that if all the replies were arranged, they would constitute an excellent review of the whole anemia problem. These letters did not all come from physicians in small towns; the folders include correspondence with other professors who wanted specific information about some interesting and important point.

A United States Senator wrote about his son, and George replied:

> I am indeed sorry to learn of your son's illness, and I do wish that I could write you that we know some way to cure chronic myelogenous leukemia. I feel sure that in the Naval Hospital at Bethesda there are excellent people who are well acquainted with this disease and its treatment. One of these is a young man whom I trained here, Lt. Commander Eugene M. Lozner. I would give anything if I could tell you that there is some new form of treatment that is worthwhile. I do wish I could write you in a more optimistic vein.

A doctor in Maine was very appreciative of the help in Dr. Minot's letter and sent him a present, which Dr. Minot acknowledged:

> Truly you are very thoughtful and kind, but there is no need for you to send me a check for my answering simple questions for you. If you had wanted me to study blood preparations by mail and critically evaluate the record of the past, so that it would be in the nature of a consultation and therefore occupied some period of time, it might then have been appropriate for me to have received a small check. I return the check because I really do not feel that it is proper for me to accept it for simply answering your letter.

Correspondence concerning publications increased and he complained: "One of the difficulties I find in this organization is that the men are constantly being asked to write what I call 'Review' or 'Rehash' articles, and it becomes difficult for them to constantly write such articles and also to produce new scientific work, or what I call 'Original Communications.'" One editor wanted Minot and Castle to write a whole book on "The Modern Diagnosis and Treatment of the Anemias for the General Practitioner." It did not take long to answer that one: "Absolutely impossible. We are hopelessly crowded with manuscript work. Whereas we have thought about this matter before, we will not be able to do anything about it for two years at the shortest."

When in 1927 his friend, Dr. Russell L. Cecil of New York, proposed that a new *Text-Book of Medicine* be published,[1] with each disease to be described in simple terms by the man best qualified to do it, he thought it was a fine idea, and he agreed to be responsible for the writing of several of the sections concerned with diseases of the blood. He revised his chapters for each new edition, including the seventh, which was published in 1947. Dr. Cecil's secretary had not a little trouble in persuading George to complete his manuscripts before the deadline.

The Macmillan Company wanted his help and advice in publishing a series of "Medical Monographs," and they wanted him to be editor of the series. George knew very well which subjects needed a thorough review and study, and he knew which authors were best qualified to write about them. The trouble was that many of these prospective authors were just like him, "hopelessly busy," and that meant still more correspondence. The Macmillan folder measures one and three quarter inches in thickness!

In the years between 1935 and 1940, the whole field of medicine was undergoing another change. When George and I had graduated in 1912, the total expenditures of the Harvard Medical School came to about three hundred thousand dollars. In 1935, the figure was almost up to twelve hundred thousand, or four times as much, the increase due in large measure to the cost of research. One of the things that always appealed to George was the constant effort to raise the standards of medical practice in the country as a whole. In April 1935, the Board of Regents of the American College of Physicians, meeting in Philadelphia, voted to organize the American Board of Internal Medicine, with nine members — six to be appointed by the College and three to be appointed by the Section on the Practice of Medicine of the American Medical Association. The Board proposed to pass on the qualifications of all those who wanted to be considered as "Specialists in Internal Medicine," and to grant a certificate when the criteria were fulfilled. To start the scheme, all the members of certain national medical societies were certified at once *ipso facto,* but after that it was ruled that certification must depend upon the ability to pass comprehensive examinations, and to show evidence of good moral character. George approved this plan, but not all the full-time professors did approve. At Johns Hopkins it was voted "to go on record as opposing the principle that certification . . . shall be made a condition of appointment or promotion . . . ." In the twenty years of its existence, the Board has become well established, and most of the young graduates who plan to work in internal medicine take the examinations for certification — the "American Boards" — in addition to the "National Boards," which give them the legal right to practice medicine in most of the states.

Around 1935, the American Foundation, Inc. transferred its activity from the field of international law to studies of the relation of government to trade, to communication, and finally to health. The procedure followed was to present problems to competent groups and then to assemble the results of the free discussion.

The idea was new, and George was a bit skeptical. He wrote first to Dean Burwell of the Medical School: "I have a letter from Miss [Esther E.] Lape [member-in-charge]." This letter was concerned with the relation of government to the over-all problems of medical care, and George asks, "Shall I answer it? Who else has these letters, and who is taking interest in them?"

George wanted to keep himself in good company, and when he found that many of his professor friends had answered, he wrote a long letter, which included this:

> Mediocrity in medicine surrounds us; it is easy and comfortable, but also it is highly contagious. Better education for all doctors is what is needed. The much-debated questions regarding one or another sort of insurance, or State medicine, whatever that term may mean, seem to me to be "surface problems" because the basic ones of the economic social aspects of the world should be understood first. Man has much to learn about himself.

His letter must have appealed to the Foundation, for in their reply he read the suggestion that he might write a magazine story or the like, and that idea amused him. He joined the Medical Advisory Committee.

At about the same time he joined the Physicians for the Improvement of Medical Care, Inc., and signed the "Principles and Proposals," the chief Principle being that "the health of the people is a direct concern of the Government," and the chief Proposal being that public funds should be made available for medical education, for research, and for hospitals.

He talked several times with his two businessmen brothers about the economics of medical care. He liked the idea of government subsidies for medical education and research, but he was very much afraid that the grant of public money might be accompanied by a restriction to the free use of that money, and he could not stand that.

In 1936, there was talk about a large hospital for the treatment of chronic diseases to be built by the Massachusetts State Depart-mentment of Health. Dr. Minot, thinking mostly of chronic arthritis, wrote to the Commissioner's Assistant-in-charge:

> Before the building is planned, two things are needed — men and a budget. Success will depend on the superior quality of the minds of the staff and the freedom and tranquility permitted them . . . The original group and the leaders of the staff might well continue to serve as a professional council . . . The active demonstration of the care of the patient and the investigation of his problems will determine just what are the needs of the estimated 138,000 individuals with chronic rheumatism in Massachusetts, and how they can best be met with the least expense.

He knew that his recommendations were a bit idealistic for a new development to be established by the State government, but still he felt bound to present them. The Lemuel Shattuck Hospital at Forest Hills, costing $16,000,000 was opened in September 1954.

In the fall of 1936 George was made Chairman of the Faculty Committee on the Harvard Medical School Library. He was glad of the appointment, for he was always interested in the history of medicine and in the part that men of Harvard had played in it. He was sensitive to their achievements and had a strong desire to maintain their high standards of accomplishment. He was very proud of his medical heritage. Browsing among old books had made him see the wisdom of his predecessors and the similarity of their problems to his own. As the Medical School had grown, each new department had collected its own small library of books, but so maintained it that it was difficult to know where any particular book might be. The need for a large centralized library became imperative, and about 1913 several rooms on the first floor of the Administration Building were taken over for the library, to the great satisfaction of both Faculty and students.

When the Harvard School of Public Health was organized in 1922, the decision to make its special collection a part of the central library was wise, and in 1928 the library was moved again, this time to the second floor of the Administration Building, which was remodeled to provide stacks and two large reading rooms.

Today the central library has about 110,000 volumes, and, even more important, it has a copy of the Union Catalogue, which lists all the incunabula, the books, and the journals held by the Boston Medical Library in its own building at 22 The Fenway and by the libraries owned by several of the hospitals in Boston. "Since," as Miss Anna Holt, the very competent librarian, says, "the generosity in making loans to its neighbors is unlimited," each individual library has access to the books in every other library. In a sense, therefore, there is only one medical library in Boston, and the combined collection is not surpassed by either the Library of the Surgeon General in Washington or the Library of the Academy of Medicine in New York.

Although George was Chairman of the Library Committee for only one year, his interest in the Library continued all his life. He sent to Miss Holt at frequent intervals "great piles of all kinds of material received at his home and office," so that she could sort it over, to keep some and dispose of the rest. Often, a most unusual item would be slipped in "just for the fun of it." Such items were always recognized and acknowledged by Miss Holt, apparently to George's considerable satisfaction, because more of the same always followed. Postcards and notes on old scraps of paper or old-book catalogue covers came almost daily, inquiring whether the Library had such an item — "If not, you should have." And often he would add, "If you have not the money to buy it let me know, because I have a small fund to use for such a purpose. Order it, if you want it." This method applied not alone to old material of historical interest, but many times to expensive new publications.

His fund was a small memorial gift, which had been given to him personally by a grateful patient to be used for the Library. This fund gave him great pleasure; he liked to buy books, preferably the interesting old items. He loved to browse in bookshops, especially in the old-book department, and when secondhand books were displayed on the street, he would linger over them to make sure that some important item was not included inadvertently. His friend, Mrs. Augustus P. Loring, had told him once that she had seen an interesting cover quite loose by itself in a great jumble of books on the table in a secondhand store. There was something about that cover that excited her, and she kept searching through the whole mess until at last she found the book itself, with the back cover that matched. It turned out to be a valuable first edition, and when the binding was repaired, she was offered fifty dollars for her investment of twenty-five cents, but she did not take it. George always remembered her story.

For some years, George had been coming over to the office at 311 Beacon Street on one or two afternoons a week to see private patients in consultation. This gave him a chance to examine people who were well-to-do and whose mode of life was different from that of most of the hospital ward patients and to give them the benefit of his superior knowledge. Most of these private patients had been seen in advance of the appointment with the Chief by one of the Junior men — Dr. George P. Reynolds, Dr. Richard B. King, or Dr. Richard P. Stetson. When the preliminary studies, including x-rays and laboratory tests, did not show any abnormality and the patient was still suffering from aches and pains in various parts, then it was Dr. Minot who could unravel the complexities of the hectic life and demonstrate that the symptoms depended upon a general cause which was not so complicated after all. There are not a few people today who owe their good health and their general happiness to the changes in their outlook on life and in their daily habits that followed from the explanation and the advice that Dr. George Minot gave them, after he had convinced himself that no underlying disease was holding them down.

There were, of course, many other patients who were sent in because of his special knowledge. Some came from as far away as California to learn the latest information about leukemia or Hodgkin's disease, or about pernicious anemia itself. One can be sure that after the careful study by the "Master" and his assistants, they went away with a clearer idea of their problem. They learned the new "tricks" in treatment and the fallacies of elaborate procedures that read well on paper but have no support in laboratory tests. Best of all, they learned from his own example the art of living courageously in spite of a serious handicap.

On September 1, 1935, Dr. Locke, the mainstay of the "firm"

at 311 Beacon Street, resigned from his hospital appointment and retired from his considerable private practice to take charge of student health at Williams College. George wrote him: "A truly sad event happened at midnight, August 31 — namely, the 'firm' of Locke and Minot ceased to exist. [The faithful associates, Drs. Blake, Reynolds, King, and Stetson, were taken for granted.] It is simply beyond my command of words to describe what it means to me to be left alone at 311 and at the City Hospital. All are younger than I at both places." In 1936, business at 311 was not good. It was beginning to be hard to pay the expenses of the office, and George worried about it. He missed the guiding hand of his friend Locke.

This lack of business is interesting. Here was an outstanding physician, who had just received the highest honor that the world can bestow. He had demonstrated his love for people, his ability to take excellent care of his patients, his devotion to his duty. He had three assistants, each an able doctor who had his own following of patients. The work at 311 was done well, and it was very effective.

Why should there be any difficulty? One would suppose that doctors all over the country would be clamoring to send their troublesome problem-patients to such an office, where the chance of accurate appraisal and sound advice would seem to be so good. What did Dr. Locke have or what did he do that made the "firm" so successful in its beginning?

These are good questions. The reason why one doctor is more successful than another, in spite of equal education and experience, is said to depend on personality, and yet George had plenty of that! One can say that he was too busy to come to the office more than once or twice a week, and that his patients saw much more of the assistants than they saw of him. The fact of the matter is that if George Minot had really wanted more business, he could have had it. In 1936, he did not care to have it.

In June 1935, he gave the ninth Alpha Omega Alpha Lecture at the annual meeting of this honorary undergraduate society. His paper was so good that it was subsequently published in the *Journal of the American Medical Association.*[2] Here are a few sentences:

> Much time has been wasted by men attempting things for which they have neither qualifications nor training. The diagnosis of the person is too often neglected, while the diagnosis of the case is made in detail . . .

Many people may walk through fields and woods and see nothing, while others may see every conceivable activity of plants, insects, and birds . . .

One cannot train a clinical investigator by any rule of thumb . . .

At that time, George was on many committees. At Harvard, he was on the Committee on Admission, on the Committee on Admission of Students to Advanced Standing, and on the Committee on Fellowships. He was on the Faculty Council, on the Administrative Board, and on the Executive Committee of the Department of Medicine. He liked this kind of thing; it kept him in contact with the affairs of the Medical School. He was always inquisitive about what was going on and who was making it go — and, since he did know so much about so many things, and especially about so many people, his advice contributed to the effectiveness of each committee. So many committee meetings, however, took his time and strength, and there were those, like Soma Weiss, who wanted him to give up some of his commitments. It was suggested that he might give up the Medical Library, but George complained: "Don't they realize that I get much pleasure and relaxation in looking at catalogues, in browsing through old books, and that it is no great trouble for me to send a note or two to Miss Holt from time to time? I do not want to give it up at all."

In the spring of 1936, Marian came down with mumps, and a few days later the children caught the disease. On the next day, George himself developed mumps and was miserable at home for nearly three weeks. His "sugar machinery" was disturbed by the infection, and his blood sugar rose to over 300 milligrams. "This losing a month of time disturbs me, and the more I worry about it, the worse I feel," he said. As usual, however, the confinement gave him a chance to enjoy his library.

When he had recovered, he went to Toronto, where he had a pleasant time and talked well. On the way back he stopped over to give talks in Cambridge and in Gloversville, New York, and two talks in Albany. He was tired when he got home, but later he wrote to Dr. Joslin: "These are pleasing days — I feel better and stronger — can walk farther before my legs will pain again."

For nine summers, up until 1935, the Minots had spent at least a month at Northeast Harbor in the cottage in the fir trees near the harbor entrance. In 1933 they had varied the program by chartering the schooner *Astrea* from their cousin, Mr. W. Rodman Peabody, for three weeks. In that lovely boat they made a cruise from Rockland to Passamaquoddy Bay and back with their daughter Marian, then aged fifteen, and their cousins the Chadwicks.

The eastern extremity of the Maine Coast and that part of New Brunswick that touches on Passamaquoddy Bay always had a fascination for George. His cruises in the *Dorel* to New Brunswick had been the high light of the season. Now he was delighted to show Marian the beauties of Roque Island, of Cutler, and of Head Harbor on Campobello. He sent me a postcard showing where the *Astrea* was anchored one night, well into the mouth of the Magaguadavic River, where he could throw a stone onto land in almost every direction.

After 1936, Mount Desert Island was getting too crowded and "swell" for George and Marian, and so they went to North Haven, Maine, where life was much more simple and natural for them. The thoroughfare that separates two islands is a beautiful stretch of water. Summer people live on both sides of it, and that means that sailing is a necessity as well as a pleasure. The little town is at the place where the thoroughfare curves and widens a little to make a landlocked harbor with east and west entrances. The Casino Wharf is the center of activities, being near the post office, the general store, and the market. In some years the Minots lived in one of the Casino flats; in others they rented one of the summer cottages. Both George and Marian loved North Haven almost as much as Northeast, especially as many old friends from Boston were on hand to love it with them. They purchased the *Marel,* one of the class of "Herreshoff Twelves," sometimes called "Dough Dishes," a corruption of "Duodici," the Italian word for twelve. They are beautifully designed and built little boats with jib and mainsail rig and a lead keel which make them ideal for children to learn to sail. George and Marian liked to sail the *Marel* around the harbor, and they were delighted when the children took part in the races and came home with a pennant or two. As usual, however, the main activity was the expeditions, sometimes in the *Marel* but more often in a motor boat, to some lovely isolated spot where the children could swim and all could have a delicious picnic lunch. Except during the war years,

George and Marian went to the Coast of Maine every summer until 1946.

In September 1936, Harvard University celebrated the three-hundredth anniversary of its founding with impressive academic ceremonies. During the week before the Tercentenary itself, a series of conferences were held on many aspects of the arts and sciences, and on the Monday and Tuesday of "The Week," beginning September 14, four symposia were held at the Medical School, each presided over by a distinguished Harvard authority in the area under discussion, the subjects and the chairmen being: "Nutrition," Professor George Richards Minot; "The Nervous System," Professor Walter Bradford Cannon; "Infectious Diseases," Professor Hans Zinsser; and "The Endocrines," Professor James Howard Means. Comparable meetings were held by the Harvard Dental School and the School of Public Health. George's Chairman's Address, "Harvard and Nutrition," was scholarly.

Back in 1934 in Copenhagen, George had met Professor Hagedorn, who was in charge of one of the two government laboratories making insulin in Denmark. Dr. Hagedorn had been working on the problem of making the effect of a single injection of insulin last much longer, and at last he had learned how to combine insulin with a protamine substance of low solubility containing zinc. Protamine zinc insulin was relatively new, but Dr. Joslin wanted to try it on George. Unfortunately it did not work very well.

On January 5, 1937, George wrote to Dr. Joslin:

> Protamine was begun on December 23. One horribly poor time ever since. Very disagreeable days with reactions, odd symptoms, and bright red sugar tests. Quite unable to tell what I can do day to day, and I am hopelessly backed up in every aspect of work. Lectures ahead and a great many duties. Residents I have not laid eyes on for weeks — and so the pessimistic story goes. I have felt I ought to quit about all I do, sell this place, and retire to the country and try to act more pleasantly. I will plan to see you and pour forth a long tale of woe at the end of this week.

He said more than this to Dr. Locke in Williamstown, and added this:

The day will come soon when I am out of it all — have to sell the house! Even so, it is pleasant to be made a member of the Saturday Club and have the privilege of talking freely and informally with such men as President Lowell, Bishop Lawrence, and Mr. Mark A. de Wolf Howe. On May 5 I am supposed to make an address at the opening of the new Mellon Institute for Industrial Research in Pittsburgh — on the same program with [Karl Taylor] Compton and [Irving] Langmuir — but not a word is written so far. I hope to see you soon so that you will cheer me up. Stetson is of the greatest comfort to me and Fitz is very helpful too, but Joslin is annoying in making me keep on with this protamine stuff when he can see that it upsets me no end.

Meantime, we have appointed some nice new men to the Thorndike, and if only I had the time and strength to give to them, we could all take advantage of the opportunity . . . In February I talk to the National Social Workers Association, and I must collect my thoughts on that.

In the spring he began to have trouble with his eyes. There was blurring of vision and dizziness at times. Dr. Paul Chandler examined him carefully but could find no direct effect of the diabetes on the eye, and considered a muscle spasm of some sort. New glasses were prescribed, and later still different glasses, but they did not seem to make much difference. Each visit took much longer than for the ordinary patient. On account of his bad legs and his reactions, and now his eyes, he gave up smoking entirely in 1937.

And then comes a fact that is always of interest. No matter whether the disease is peptic ulcer or chronic headaches or arthritis or asthma or even diabetes, as soon as the victim can get away to a place that is attractive to him, his symptoms improve rapidly. That summer up in North Haven, Maine, all was well again. The protamine zinc insulin interlude had been quite forgotten.

Another event in 1937 was the visit of the Nylins from Sweden. Dr. Gustav Nylin was a distinguished physician, interested primarily in diseases of the heart. When the Minots had gone to Sweden, Dr. Paul D. White had written to Dr. Nylin to introduce the Minots, and at the meeting the Nylins had been most cordial and hospitable to the Minots. After the exchange of hospitality, George corresponded with Dr. Nylin.

When a Professorship of Medicine at Oxford had been offered to Dr. Castle, George's emotions had been somewhat mixed. Although he was most gratified to think that his right-hand man was good enough to be considered for such an important post, he knew full well that Castle's departure would be disastrous for the Thorndike, and George wrote to Dr. Nylin: "Castle got back from Oxford on June 30. I am delighted to tell you that he has refused the Oxford offer and is to stay at the Thorndike with a promotion to a full Professorship. This pleases me very much . . ."

On December 24, 1937, he wrote again:

> I shall, of course, be interested to learn what arrangements are made for the medical professorships that are open in Stockholm . . . Of course to my way of thinking, Dr. Nylin should receive one of the vacant posts. Have you heard that Witts has accepted the Nuffield Professorship at Oxford, the position Castle turned down.

In another letter to Dr. Nylin, in October 1938, George said:

> It was certainly most kind of you and Mrs. Nylin to give Dr. Weiss such a delightful time when he was in Stockholm . . . On October 10 the Harvard Corporation confirmed the appointment of Dr. Weiss as Professor of Medicine as of September 1, 1939. He is to take Dr. Christian's place at the Brigham Hospital, and we are thus assured that that clinic will develop in splendid fashion. You can realize that it is upsetting to Dr. Castle, Keefer and myself to have Weiss leave here . . . What is the gossip about making appointments in your part of the world?

Still later, he wrote:

> Castle has been back a week and of course he had a remarkable experience seeing the world . . . Next Saturday, December 10, I have been asked to speak for three minutes on the radio regarding the significance of the Nobel Prize . . . how it acted to bring together individuals in different countries, because . . . science and literature are not bounded by international borders.

During the winter of 1937–38 Cousin Jim was not at all well. In the summer, he had been hospitalized with a severe respiratory infection, and had come out only fairly well. George had worried about him, but Dr. Stetson had not found anything wrong other than that his years were beginning to tell. During the winter, the old gentleman was coughing, and was quite short of breath, but, even so, George had not hesitated to keep his own speaking dates at the Mayo Clinic and at the University of Minnesota.

In late April 1938, George took his wife and his daughter Marian on a trip planned to include several meetings, ending with the meeting of the Association of American Physicians, of which George was then President, in Atlantic City. The first stop was Washington, where George made his first attendance following his election to the National Academy of Sciences. In Richmond, he gave the two Stuart McGuire Lectures in Medicine at the Medical College of Virginia, and it was after the second, when he had hardly sat down, that a telegram was handed to him bearing the news that his father had taken a turn for the worse and was critically ill. George and the two Marians had somewhat less than an hour in which to pack their things and catch the night train. Cousin Jim died before they arrived in Boston.

After the funeral, George felt lonely. The death of one's father always means a break with the past — the crossing of a bar without possibility of return. "I feel as if I had grown ten years older, being now the oldest of my immediate family and near relatives," he wrote in a little note to me.

Cousin Jim's death meant that George could not go to Atlantic City to take his place as President of the Association of American Physicians. He had prepared for the meeting so well, however, and had considered and settled in advance so many of the little problems, that the Secretary, Dr. Hugh J. Morgan, and the Vice President, Dr. Eugene F. Dubois, had little trouble in carrying on; but the "telephone wires were kept hot arranging for the last-minute details," as George said. After the meeting Dr. Morgan wrote to him, "You are the only President since I have taken office as Secretary who really took over the running of the Association from the time of your election . . . Under the circumstances, things went off very well, thanks to your thoughtfulness."

George's Presidential Address[3] was read for him by Dr. Dubois, who presided. It was, in essence, an analysis of the past programs of the Association, and in it several interesting facts appeared. There had been no papers on typhoid fever since 1935. Tuberculosis as a cause of death had decreased markedly, but the study of its mechanism was still a problem, as was shown by the number of papers concerned with it on every program. Interest in diseases of the heart and blood vessels had doubled in twenty years; and this was a conservative conclusion, because it did not consider the formation of several special organizations for those interested in heart disease, and the numerous papers presented at these special meetings.

Cancer [George wrote] now stands second only to heart disease as a cause of death in this country . . . It is apt to be thought of as a condition to be studied and discussed by surgeons and radiologists, and this probably accounts in part for the relatively few papers on the subject [at these meetings of physicians] . . . The problem of cancer will probably not be solved by surgical or radiological procedures, and eventually I suspect may be treated or prevented by so-called medical measures.

The following remarks were part of what he said on his favorite topic:

The falling off of communications concerning physiologic alterations of the nervous systems or so-called functional disorders is particularly striking . . . [and yet] such problems are of increasing importance . . . A considerable fraction of the successful care and treatment of patients, and undoubtedly the prevention of much illness, is to be identified with the proper consideration of social, psychological, and allied factors . . . The doctor . . . must have an understanding of the problems of human beings.

After the meeting many members wrote George letters of sympathy and regret that he had been detained by such a sad circumstance. Dr. Dubois was particularly solicitous and was kind enough to suggest that in 1939, when he himself would be President, George must preside on the first day. This was very pleasing, and George accepted, but added a characteristic bit: "I would like to suggest, however, that as your President's Address will come first on the first day . . . you would be good enough to preside until the middle of the morning. As you probably know, my metabolic behavior is such that I never do things very well until an hour and a half after breakfast."

In May 1938 came a letter of another kind — a registered letter from London informing George that he had been elected a Fellow of the Royal College of Physicians (London). He wrote to his brother Jimmy about this, saying: "One never knows about ones relatives unless they give information . . . Since 1931 I have been a Fellow of the Royal College of Physicians *Edinburgh* but the London organization is the more significant . . . Now I can write

F.R.C.P. (Lond.) after my name . . . Papa, I know, would have been pleased with the Londoners' action." And he adds: "A year ago I was elected to the National Academy of Sciences (of America). There are 6 M.D.'s that are members."

George was always interested in the postgraduate education of doctors. In June 1938, the Council of the Massachusetts Medical Society agreed to sponsor a clinical congress or assembly. George was much interested in this Assembly; he served on the Program Committee, but did not present a paper.

The autumn of 1939 was an anxious time for the whole world. The news from overseas became more dreadful and made America restless. A letter from George's friend, Professor Gunnar Holmgren, a little later, was concerned with the difficulties of printing the Scandinavian journals: "The Russian airforce is likely to destroy the presses . . . In Finland, fighting against many times superior Russian forces, the expressions of sympathy from the whole world have made a strong impression, and more active help of different kinds starts coming from various quarters — airplanes from Italy, and Finnish-Americans in the U.S.A. and volunteers, especially from Sweden, are gathering in quite big numbers. Let us hope that the help does not arrive too late."

George answered promptly: "My chief thoughts are for all the people in the Scandinavian countries. Words utterly fail to express the way we feel here, and we send our sincere sympathies."

All through the Battle of Britain he kept up a steady correspondence with Dr. Janet Vaughan. She wrote later, "His letters were a bright light in a dark place . . . They showed again that Great Britain had friends, and I had a distinguished friend."

In late 1939, our classmate, Dr. Philip D. Wilson, had offered to lead an orthopedic unit to Britain, and he asked George to serve on his Medical Advisory Board to help in choosing good doctors and raising money for the Allied Relief Fund. George was delighted to lend his name and to help as much as possible.

There were other activities in 1939. Dr. William S. Middleton has described for me "The Symposium on the Blood" which was held that year in Madison, Wisconsin. "A group of students of the subject, including [Louis K.] Diamond, [Einar] Meulengracht [of

Denmark], [Edward B.] Krumbhaar, [Cecil J.] Watson, [Russell L.] Haden and others constituted one of the most distinguished gatherings of scientists that this campus has ever entertained. Dr. Minot was the lodestone; and wherever he stopped, a group of his admirers gathered. I never saw him in better form, nor more effective." And then Dr. Middleton adds another bit:

"Dr. Charles H. Bunting, long-time Professor of Pathology in the University of Wisconsin Medical School . . . [had an] interest in the cytologic aspects of hematology [which] gave him close rapport with Dr. Minot. Miss Ethel Thewlis, skilled technician in hematology, is still with us in the University Hospitals. The period that she spent with Dr. Minot has brought double dividends to her and to the University of Wisconsin Medical School. We shall be ever indebted to him for his painstaking guidance of Miss Thewlis during the Boston period."

At the Thorndike in September 1939, conditions were more difficult. Two key men were to be lost at the same time. Dr. Soma Weiss was called to the Brigham, and although Dr. Chester S. Keefer was ready and qualified to take his place, it was only a year later that Keefer in turn was offered and accepted the Wade Professorship of Medicine at Boston University. These men were at the head of an impressive list of "Thorndike men" who were chosen by many medical schools to become their new Professors of Medicine. The original selection of intelligent, attractive men, the atmosphere of open and friendly discussion and mutual cooperation, and the insistence upon accomplishment were the three principles which Francis Peabody and George Minot had carried out, and now the results were demonstrated.

From the opening of the Thorndike in the autumn of 1923 to George Minot's resignation in 1949, there had been something over four hundred young doctors who had served in the institution for longer or shorter periods as resident physicians or as research fellows. It is impressive to find that among the "graduates" there are today thirty-eight professors of medicine or of pediatrics and five professors of medical science like chemistry or bacteriology. There are twenty-two associate professors and four assistant professors. From the Harvard Medical Unit at the Boston City Hospital, outside of the Thorndike Memorial Laboratory itself, have come twenty-five other men who hold high academic positions in medicine, including ten full professorships. In addition, there is a list of sixteen distinguished foreign physicians who have worked at the Thorndike.

This makes a total of 110 doctors important in medicine who received a part of their training in the Harvard Medical Unit, including the Thorndike Memorial Laboratory, at the Boston City Hospital. These men — and there are three women too — are now working in various parts of the world: in Australia, China, Peru, and South Africa, as well as in Belgium, Britain, and Holland. Very recently Dr. George Packer Berry, present Dean of the Harvard Medical School, has written: "The contribution which the Thorndike has made to American Medicine [he might have said World Medicine] is truly impressive . . . [these men] are the 'living shadows' of great teachers such as Francis Peabody, George Minot, Soma Weiss and their successors." [4]

Each time that George talked on the radio, it was for him an important event. What he would say had to be written out with the greatest care so that the wording would be exactly correct, and then he practiced the reading of it to his wife to be sure that he would sound natural and at ease. In 1940, Dr. C. C. Little, who had been with George in the early days at the Huntington Hospital and was now president of the American Society for the Control of Cancer, had asked him to give a broadcast on the curability of cancer. George seized the opportunity to discuss the need for more critical investigations of the physiological aspects, and he added a word about the importance of a medical education that would produce physicians who were well trained and who could approach the problem with a broad perspective.

In 1941 the Massachusetts Medical Society and the Massachusetts State Department of Health had been joint sponsors of a series of radio talks called "Green Lights to Health," and George talked again on cancer, this time on its prevention, and his emphasis was on the need for thorough examination of the individual by competent doctors.

When he was asked to lecture to the Association for Research in Nervous and Mental Disease on "The Problems of Nutritional Deficiency," the title pleased him because it was not limited to vitamin deficiencies, and he could talk about food in general, including the pleasures of eating under proper circumstances. Perhaps he thought of the remark he had made to the newspaper reporter as he sailed to Europe, about the "pastry and chocolate milk shake" diet of stenographers. There was an amusing item about this particular talk, for he wrote the Chairman, "I notice that you have me down as the first speaker. As I think you know, there is a rule that I never speak before 10:30 A.M. If you can iron out that difficulty, I will see what I can do."

George was always solicitous about his house officers and residents. To a successful candidate he wrote, after congratulating him, "Please enjoy your vacation and forget all about medicine. Come back refreshed to proceed with your work."

One of his former students, whom George had invited to become one of his residents, said that he would prefer to go to the Massachusetts General Hospital, if he could get in. Instead of being annoyed by the man's refusal, George wrote a good letter, which probably helped the student to be accepted by the M.G.H. When, later on, George saw the man's name on a list of those who had been appointed, he wrote him a short note of congratulation.

Another student pleased him very much, chiefly because his thesis showed that he had learned his lesson well. Under the title of "The Vanishing Patient," the thesis told why Amado, the guitar player with a history of several hemorrhages from his stomach, had escaped from the hospital and run home. First, he had been badly frightened by all that was done to him in the first few days, including x-rays and blood studies of all kinds. Second, everyone had been interested in his case, but no one doctor had been in charge or had taken the trouble to explain to him what this interest was all about. Third, there was no attempt to study him as a person or to examine the conditions at his home. The thesis concludes: "It is only when we have a careful blending of the person with his social situation and with his medical care that we can expect success in treatment. If we do not have this, we have a Vanishing Patient." George was delighted.

In 1941, George was pleased to "find" Dr. Charles Sprecher

Davidson. Like Dr. Hale Ham, he was an attractive, bright, intelligent young man with new ideas and the desire to test them. He came from California, by way of McGill University Medical School and an internship at the San Francisco Hospital, to be Assistant Resident at the Thorndike. He has been there ever since, still devoted to Dr. Minot's memory and to the work on the diseases of the blood. Meantime, he has become Associate Professor of Medicine in the Harvard Medical School, and he is a Special Consultant to the section on Biochemistry and Nutrition of the United States Public Health Service. George chose well.

George was anxious to have each of his men prepare at least one paper for one or another meeting of the American Society for Clinical Investigation — the "young Turks" — in Atlantic City. He was very particular about the wording. "Look here," he would say, "you can do better than that! Take it home and read it to your wife, and you will see how to make it read smoother and easier. I am sure that you can cut out some of the words to shorten and sweeten the whole thing. Remember that you are allowed only ten minutes in which to present the results of your year's work. Ask yourself what it is that you want to put across and then put just that. Be careful of your language. It is not *cases* who are disabled, it is *patients* — that is to say *people* — who are disabled. It is not the gallstone which suffers the pain, it is the patient who has the stone."

After George died, Dr. Janet Vaughan wrote to Marian:

> I count it always as my greatest richness that I worked at the Thorndike in its most active days, and that I was trained to work by such a scholar as George Minot.
>
> Two days before I was to read a paper at Atlantic City, I showed him the notes I was to use. A blue pencil went through them all because of imperfections of style . . . [He wanted] the meaning crystal clear, the English to his liking . . . He rehearsed us all with much personal advice before we read a paper to the learned society. Whatever work we have done since then has instinctively been measured against his standards.

A similar letter came from Dr. A. B. Meikeljohn, another English visitor, who wrote:

> His industry was amazing. Besides the Thorndike Memorial Laboratory, he played a prominent part in the direction of the Harvard Medi-

cal School. Yet he found time to read and annotate with marginal notes a great variety of medical journals. Often his staff would find on their desks on Monday morning a scrap of paper drawing their attention to a recent article which they should have found for themselves but had not. His own room in the Thorndike, with its library of journals and the fellowship diplomas of the British Royal Colleges hung on the walls, was constantly open to his staff, and in looking up a reference one was often rewarded by finding a marginal comment by G.R.M. expressing his views on its merit. He believed strongly that a medical scientist should be aware of developments in fields of science outside his own specialty and even outside of medicine, and this was a discipline which he firmly imposed on himself. His advocacy of social medicine was disturbing to some of his contemporaries.

He was a master of detail. No letter went unanswered, and if a note from him was not acknowledged in twenty-four hours, it was usually followed by another asking if the first had been received.

His secretary was once handed a notice to put up on the [bulletin] board. A pencilled spot at the top of the paper surrounded by a circle was indicated by an arrow from a written directive: "Put thumbtack here."

A member of his staff, having made an appointment to see him, would often be greeted by the production of his watch. "Now, let's see," he would say, "I can give you just 45 seconds. No, let's say, at a guess, a minute and 15 seconds." An hour later the young man would emerge, his head dizzy with the wide range of topics that had been brought to his attention.[6]

Loose papers, without titles, names, or dates, troubled him. "The lack of any label is careless and sloppy," he said. "It doesn't take long to write a name and a date, does it?"

He was always delighted with my story about Dr. Longcope in New York because he agreed so heartily with its principles. One afternoon Dr. Longcope came into the laboratory just as I had finished the all-day job of making an extract of horse dander to test for horse asthma. When he picked up the tube of straw-colored fluid, he said:

"H'm, it looks like ordinary culture broth, doesn't it? What is in this next tube?"

"That's the broth," I said.

"How do you tell which is which?"

When I explained that the extract was in the left-hand tube and that it had a slightly darker color, he was neither pleased nor satisfied.

"Look here!" he said. "You will use this material for important tests on patients, and all the while you will never be quite certain of what it is. I am going to pour the contents of both tubes in the sink. Tomorrow will you please begin all over again and make a new extract, and this time *for God's sake, label your tubes!"* — and Dr. Longcope did not often swear.

In June 1943, Miss Curtis retired and George engaged a new secretary, Miss Anne M. Bement, the daughter of a classmate, and a bright girl. She remembers several high lights.

One was his return from lunch:

> Usually he returned about 2:30 P.M., but his moods varied, from telling us of a strange bird he had just seen, to inquiring who a girl was he had just passed in the hall, to coming in with four fingers on each hand crossed and saying, "Don't say anything until I tell you these things I want to remember!" And, unwrapping each finger, he would relate the eight items that were to be remembered. He never forgot why he crossed his fingers, and the other people in the Thorndike came to respect the crossed fingers — no one spoke to him until they had been uncrossed and a notation made of the data contained in each finger.
>
> Dr. Minot's memory for the place of each book in his rows of ceiling-high bookcases was phenomenal. He knew where each book belonged and exactly what position in the case it had. It was not an uncommon incident to be taking dictation about an appointment for a patient, or the like, when a look of horror would come on his face. "My God, it's gone, someone's stolen it, where is it?" Not having any idea what was gone, what was stolen, or where it was, we would ask what "it" was. We found as he would rise to his feet and go to the bookcase, mumbling to himself about filing a claim with the insurance company for the loss of such a valuable book, that one of his medical books was missing. "My God, here it is, down on the fifth shelf when it should be on the third next to Osler's *Medicine*. Now who would do something like that?" And with that crisis taken care of, he would return to his desk, calm, cool, and serene, and say, "and now, where was I in the letter to Mrs. Smith?"
>
> He was never too busy to inquire from us both [secretaries] sincerely as to our health. I shall never forget his sending me home on a Wednesday afternoon with a head cold, and telling me to stay there Thursday. On Thursday morning, at an hour when I knew he was usually his busiest, he called me on the telephone to say that he had been thinking about me and decided it was best for me to stay out until Monday so

that I could go to my family on the Cape. I assured him I would be all right on Friday, but he insisted that I not return until Monday, and when Dr. Minot made up his mind, it was for good and all and there would be no changing it. I stayed out until Monday.[7]

As has been said, one important secret of George Minot's success was his ability to choose good men. To do this, he had a knack of learning from other chiefs of departments, his friends in other schools, who their good men were and what they were going to do after graduation. There was a good reason for enjoying what others might call "gossip," for if a man was well recommended George lost no time in asking others about him, and he might even try to meet the candidate in person, in case he too was in Atlantic City. It is not surprising that he could write to the Council about the new candidates: "I feel as if I knew something about almost every man who has been nominated for 'the Society.' "

He could appraise his own undergraduate medical students easily and accurately. "G—— is an exceedingly capable student. It has given me pleasure to know that he graduated Summa Cum Laude. I give him an A for the course in 'Medicine-6.' T—— is capable — he should be given a low B or possible a high C. He will make a good House Officer. R—— is a little shy: not quite as good as T——: has difficulty distinguishing what I call the important from the unimportant."

In 1942 and 1943, the medical students were going into the Army in such numbers that it was hard to find good House Officers and Residents; indeed the number of applications for entrance to the Medical School had fallen from 1200 to 225. By special arrangements, about sixty places in the Class to begin in September 1945, had been held for men to be assigned by the Army and the Navy, and Harvard had nothing to do except to accept the men that were sent by the military authorities. "Some are very good, some are pretty good, and some, unfortunately, are rather bad," George wrote. The idea was part of the effort to help the veterans to go on with their chosen work, but it was going to interfere somewhat with the instruction, since the men with inferior backgrounds would have trouble keeping up with their superior colleagues.

In the meantime, the Faculty of the Harvard Medical School had voted in April 1943 in a ratio of about five to one, and reaffirmed the decision in May 1944, to admit women, starting with the new class in September 1945. The matter had been considered more than once in times past, but in wartime the grinding necessity of finding enough capable and well-qualified students who were not going into the armed forces turned the tide. For the class beginning in September 1945, as many as fifty-two women applied, but only five were accepted.

It is needless to say that Dr. Minot was one of those who, in a rather lively discussion, spoke against the plan and voted against it both times. "Women are not strong enough to be doctors. So soon as they marry the time and money spent on their education will be lost, and only a few will be able to carry on in laboratory work, and even a smaller number in practice," he said. I remember our own conversations about the idea of women in the dissecting room, or women as house officers in the hospital, and how the intimate talks about patients, usually in the late hours of the evening, would be affected by having women present in the house officers' "flat." Since then the world has gone on, and the women as students and house officers are doing well, most of them very well. The fact is that they do not have to sit on the bed and "go over the books" any more.

Dr. Castle remembers the faculty meeting at which Dr. Minot reported that he had just been walking in the corridor of the Harvard Medical School, and as he turned a corner there was a boy medical student with his arm around a girl medical student — "and I couldn't quite find out who it was." His sense of propriety was disturbed considerably.

In the year 1940, a very interesting activity was organized for the undergraduate medical students. On April 16, 1940, the first Undergraduate Medical Assembly was held. Its aims were: (1) to make known the investigative work of their colleagues; (2) to give undergraduates an opportunity to present their problems; (3) to offer an opportunity to become acquainted with techniques and methods of investigation; and (4) to demonstrate the possibility of undergraduate investigative work.

George was impressed with this activity, for he could see that it was stimulating and instructive to students and faculty alike. It was much more effective than the old plan of the Boylston Medical

Society, which allowed a whole evening to the presentation and discussion of a single paper. More important, the Assembly was open to the whole School.

George described the Assembly to a friend:

The papers, I think, are exactly as good as those presented at the meetings of the so-called "Young Turks" in Atlantic City, and I have always been very much impressed. The program of the first year included twelve papers, and there were eighteen additional papers that were read by title, and there have been essentially that number of papers each year since. The papers were limited in time to 10 minutes each and then 5 minutes were reserved for discussion.

In 1941 the Huntington Hospital was in trouble. It did not have enough money to support all the work that the Staff wanted to do. Professor E. B. Wilson, of the Harvard School of Public Health, declared that as much as $3,000,000 would be necessary if cancer was to be studied adequately, and, furthermore, even if the money were provided, it should be distributed among several laboratories. "There was no more reason for a special hospital for cancer than for special hospitals for arthritis or for diabetes," he said, "and quite on the contrary, the work should be done in a general hospital where the approach would be from a broad base."

But others did not agree with this theory. Dr. E. D. Churchill wrote to President Conant of Harvard: "I know only too well of the difficulties — nevertheless, I find that the course of action outlined by Professor Wilson destroys so completely the hope of realizing the very real contributions that the University might make to the cancer problem, that I am unwilling to share . . . any responsibility . . ." And Dr. Cornelius P. Rhoades, Director of the Sloan-Kettering Institute for Cancer Research in New York, wrote to Dr. Wilson:

American Medicine has progressed largely because of a single basic principle — that the segregation of patients with one type of disease in small closely integrated institutions equipped with special research facilities is sound. This was the principle upon which the hospital of the Rockefeller Institute was founded: it was Dr. [Rufus] Cole's great contribution to the advance of medical science. The most classic example is that of the Thorndike Laboratory in Boston. The Huntington closure implies that this principle is unsound and should be abandoned. I cannot believe that many would agree. For Harvard University to accept it implies that the University is willing to accept defeat [by lack of funds] and turn the clock back.

These arguments, however, were of no avail, and on November 27, 1941 *The Boston Herald* carried the headline "Harvard to Give up Noted Cancer Unit." On December 31 the Huntington was closed — that is to say, the activities of the Huntington Hospital were moved out of the building. On January 1, 1942, a whole floor of the "Domestic Building" at the Massachusetts General Hospital was given over to the Huntington staff, and new laboratories were soon in working order once more, still under the direction of Dr. Joseph C. Aub. In 1951, the Huntington laboratories were moved to occupy two floors of the new Research Building.

George was much disturbed by all this controversy. He said to me, "Goodness knows that the affairs of the School are in a tangle; we had a big argument at the Faculty meeting yesterday." He felt bad that the changes had to be made, for he agreed with Dr. Rhoades that research was more productive when it was concentrated by many people working on it together. He was interested in the Huntington Hospital not so much because he had been Chief of Medicine there as because he had seen what could be accomplished when competent workers could work together and help each other on a common problem.

13

Recognition of Authority

In April 1942, when George was fifty-six, he had an attack of herpes zoster (called also "shingles"), with skin lesions in a line around the right side of his trunk, and the poor man suffered real pain for a number of days. It was a month before the shingles cleared away. In the following June came an episode that disturbed his doctor friends. While he was talking on the telephone, there came a sudden numbness and tingling in his left arm and left leg. Since his early forties, he had had pains in his legs and feet that were "circulatory" in origin, because walking, which required more blood, made them worse. Occasional episodes of blurred vision and dizziness had also been interpreted as circulatory. The attack in June was different, because there was no paralysis or even a weakness of any muscle group; the symptoms were entirely sensory, and that led to the conclusion that the trouble was a form of neuropathy, which Dr. Joslin said was not very uncommon in diabetes. If so, the outlook was not quite so unfavorable, but it was bad enough.

All George's symptoms were very much better in the summers, when he could get away and find time to relax. In August 1942, he was up in New Hampshire. "We paddle our canoe and walk two or three miles a day," he wrote, "and some days I eat candy as a preventive of trouble [from too low blood sugar], but have had no serious reactions." Once again Dr. Joslin wanted to try protamine zinc insulin, and this time it worked much better.

As usual, Marian had been keeping her notes with great care, and her tables of figures for diet, insulin, and urine sugar can be interpreted almost at a glance. Her special reports show well the amount of work involved: "Seventy-four specimens this summer —

sixty were blue and eleven green — only three were worse than that. Since our return in September, he runs sugar most of the time."

In diabetes, the circulation in the feet is of primary importance, because if the blood supply diminishes too much, gangrene is likely to set in. George liked to sit with his shoes off and toast his feet in front of the open fire or in front of an electric sunbowl. He had sunbowls in his study downstairs and in his bedroom upstairs, and he had one in his office at the Thorndike. Of course he had been warned about the danger of burning his feet, being reminded that he did not feel heat as intensely as the normal person. He tried to be careful, of course, but the time came when he did burn his toe.

On January 5, 1943, Dr. Joslin sent him again to Dr. Leland S. McKittrick, the surgeon who had seen him in 1932. The tip of the left great toe showed a blister about 4 mm in diameter. Dr. McKittrick dressed the area at intervals, but it was not until February that healing was complete.

Six months later, in August 1943, George was up in New Hampshire once more, and he telephoned to Dr. McKittrick that he had blistered the same toe again, and in the same way. Fortunately, Dr. W. J. Paul Dye of Wolfboro was not far away, and Dr. McKittrick wrote to Dr. Dye:

> Dr. Minot has just called me up to say that he was a "damned fool" because he had a burn on his toe exactly as he had last January. There was no discussion as to his diagnosis or expression of opinion: he was right in both ways. He was lucky last January, and his toe healed up nicely in a month's time. He tells me now that there is a large blister on the toe; it is quite tense and filled with fluid.

Dr. Dye drew off the fluid, and then back in Boston Dr. McKittrick dressed the toe. It was not until November that the lesion was almost healed.

In the middle of January 1944 the pain in the feet was still present, and George was using heat as the best way of relieving it, and, sure enough, he burned his toe for a third time.

All through January and February Dr. McKittrick and Dr. F. D. Moore tried hard to heal the area, but in March it became obvious that the time had come to treat the patient and his toe intensively. George had to stay in the Deaconess Hospital for about three weeks before the toe healed. This time he had learned his lesson, and after that there was no more trouble from burns.

In spite of all these difficulties, he kept going. Gasoline was rationed in 1943, and every one of us had to be careful not to drive his car even a mile more than necessary. Like most of the doctors, George received extra points, but still not enough. Like the others, too, he and his wife learned to look ahead and try to make each trip in the car accomplish several errands at one time. In those days he could not seem to work quite so fast, but, as always, he was "hopelessly busy" and his two secretaries were busy too.

George was the typical "absent-minded professor." One night, the Medical Exchange Club dined with Dr. Enders in his apartment house. When I arrived I found George standing in the vestibule, evidently in trouble.

"How do you get into this place?" he asked. "The inside door is locked and I cannot find any bell. What will we do now?"

He had been working on the Enders mailbox, trying hard to open it, but he had missed entirely the panel of names and buttons. When I pressed the button for Dr. Enders' apartment, the loud buzzer sounded at once, and it made George jump; it really scared him.

On December 2, 1945, George was sixty years old, and on Wednesday, December 5, a birthday dinner was given in his honor at the Harvard Club of Boston.[1] Formal invitations were sent to 263 friends and colleagues in all parts of the world — to Professor Holmgren in Stockholm, and Professor Meulengracht in Copenhagen, and to other friends in England and in Europe, in South Africa and in South America.

There were seventy-two of George's friends at the dinner. Dr. Castle presided, and began this way:

"Dr. Minot, We here are among those privileged to know you personally from close association in your work. There are many others who would also like to be here to rejoice with us — those other friends and patients who knowingly or unaware owe their very lives to you."

Dr. Christian was the first speaker. He described what Harvard had meant to George, as reflected in the brilliant record of his medical school work.

Dean Burwell, on the other hand, told of what George had meant to Harvard: "He is one of the people to whom a Dean can go and know that he will look at the current problem in its relation to the whole problem — with devotion to the interests of the institution, with helpfulness, and with generosity. This is not the least of his virtues."

Dr. Castle introduced Dr. Manary as one who had known the Harvard Medical Unit at the Boston City Hospital since its inception and who had been "steadfast in his belief that the participation of the three medical schools of Boston is a great asset to the City Hospital."

Dr. Manary said: "I have been at the Boston City Hospital for 38 years and have learned that the only things worth while in life are friends . . . I am saddened by the absence of Soma Weiss." And then he said: "George Minot loves his work so much that he can play at it."

A letter from Dr. Stetson — still in the Army — was read: "After the past 45 months of destruction, it is refreshing to turn to the appreciation of one who has contributed so much."

Dr. Laurence B. Ellis pointed out "how much the world owes to Dr. Joslin for preserving the health of our Guest of Honor." And then he continued:

> The Thorndike has an atomic structure. It is unitary and indivisible . . . It is neither light weight, like hydrogen, nor inert, like lead . . . It ranks high in the scale of elements, for it gives off a constant stream of particles and rays which excite and stimulate all surrounding matter. The inner structure is a positively charged central nucleus surrounded by numerous satellites, each revolving happily in its own idiorhythmic orbit but held inexorably in its pathway by the major force emanating from the center. The nucleus has two parts: a proton heavily loaded with positive charges — known as Minot — the other, also a weighty substance, is the neutron called Castle. This neutron is in no way inert: it has positive and negative forces in such perfect balance that it is able to act as a harmonious buffer between all opposing electrical forces.
>
> The scientific history of the Thorndike will [continue] as long as the potent nuclear force at its core persists and continues to emanate its

beneficent influence not only among its multitude of scintillating satellites, but throughout the scientific world.

Dr. Joslin said, among other things: "I would like to think of your gentle, unassuming, farseeing father, once my clinical teacher, and how happy he would be if he were present on this occasion."

At that point Dr. Castle read the "Ode" that George's secretaries had written for the surprise party which they gave him on the afternoon before the birthday. On that occasion they presented him with a handsome leather desk set as a gift from all his colleagues and secretaries, both at the Thorndike and at 311.

ODE

To George Richards Minot

Written for His Sixtieth Birthday by All of His Secretaries

This is a tale of a typical day
In G.R.M.'s office, and we want to say
Our day begins at ten twenty-seven
And finds us exhausted by four eleven.

"Good Morning," he greets us, "I've too much to do;
I must see Taylor at six minutes past two;
Get Miss What's-her-name please on the phone and say
I haven't got time to make Rounds today.

"Get Tagnon to see the students for me;
I must see Williams at eleven of three.
A list is what I really need
To put in my pocket for me to read.

"I did have a list which I now have lost;
It gave some items and what they cost;
About ten or so things were on that list;
It was pink and small, and that's the gist.

"I want a list of my men; the titles they hold,
Full names and addresses, how many years old,
Their degrees, how much money they're going to get,
And where they all come from. Has Castle come yet?

"Now that our boys are coming back,
I must have a list that does not lack
What battle stars and honors they won;
The problem of which to take back has begun.

"My God, Miss Griffin, I almost forgot,
I must have a list of what Williams bought,

How much money in total has so far been spent,
Where is she, get her, I mean Miss Bement.

"There's an important person coming to see
Castle, Davidson, Taylor and me.
Have him sign in the Guest Book and please remember
We completely forgot it throughout September.

"Miss Bement, will you please sneak out and see
Who the girl in the purple dress might be?
She's down in the hall in the room on the right;
She's small with brown hair and about five feet in height.

"I'm hopelessly busy, in unusual haste,
I don't have a minute and a quarter to waste.
Now let's get going, go shut the door,
I'll speak to President Conant and not one person more.

"Has Burwell called, 'cause he said he would?
Has my Resident come? If he hasn't he should.
I'll answer the mail, though I've too much to do;
I must go to the School as soon as that's through."

At twenty-six and a half minutes past four
He's done enough and will do no more.
"We've had a hectic day," he'll say,
"Tomorrow should be easier in every way."

He puts on his coat and his hat on his head:
"I can't stop now, and as I have said,
I'll take the letters and sign them with pen
And I'll be in in the morning around about ten."

He bids us goodbye and hastens away,
And this is the end of a perfect day,
Except for the lists and the figures to get,
Which will keep us quite busy for some time yet.

We fuss and we groan and we tear our hair,
But we wouldn't change him, to this we swear;
Though we smile at his ways, we are fond of them.
Let's all drink a toast to G.R.M.

When the applause subsided, Dr. Fitz was introduced and said:

. . . Not many people realize that when Dr. Minot was a schoolboy he was a well-known naturalist, nor that his first publication . . . gives a charming and graphic account of *Melitaea gabbi* and the manner in which a *Euchloe sara* deposits an egg . . . His habits of meticulous clinical observation . . . have their roots deeply planted in another field of science.

Dr. Minot will always believe that Boston is the hub of the universe, that Harvard University is the most important center of learning in existence, and that, when speaking of hospitals, *the hospital* will always signify the Massachusetts General . . . He has a rare talent for accumulating interesting material dealing with Harvard history. One example of this talent is his "Holmes" Christmas card. Years ago there was a committee room . . . and herein was an old table with a drawer. At a certain committee meeting, while Dr. Edsall was Dean, Dr. Minot's inquisitive fingers explored the drawer, and hit upon a die which proved to be that of the admission card to Dr. Oliver Wendell Holmes' lectures on Anatomy and Physiology. It occurred to Dr. Minot to have the card reprinted and later he distributed it in the form of a Christmas card to many of his friends . . . No other of our teachers has ever been able to resurrect the past so gracefully.

Then there is the "Carmen Seculare" — a fugitive sheet of rare Harvard interest which he discovered in some obscure bookshop and presented to the Medical School library. This prints a curious song, written "in lingua Latina porcelliana," fitted to the tune of Yankee Doodle, composed by "Gulielmus Magnushumilis" and designed to be sung on the 8th of September 1836 at the celebration of the two-hundredth anniversary of the founding of Harvard College . . . Of course, "Gulielmus" means "William," "Magnus" means "Big" and "humilis" means "low" . . . and William Bigelow was . . . Phi Beta Kappa poet on two occasions. . . . The fourth and fifth stanzas, with one minor paraphrase, might have been written for this occasion . . . The translation emanates from the pen of the distinguished Latinist, E. K. Rand of the class of 1894.

Although true Puritans are shocked
  At jests that have no reason,
Old Horace claimed that it was sweet
  To play the fool in season.
And, also, wise King Solomon,
  Allotting time for sorrow,
Left proper space in all his plans
  For laughter on the morrow.

So let us all now gathered here,
  For eating and for drinking,
Sing Yankee Doodle as best we can,
  But, also, pause for thinking.
A hundred years from now, lets hope,
  May grandsons have our places;

May they enjoy as much as we
Our Minot's ample graces.

And now, Dr. Minot, I order you to rise.

When George stood up, Dr. Fitz continued:

I am directed by the President and Board of Trustees of the American Medical Association to deliver to you The Distinguished Service Medal of the Association, awarded to you for meritorious services in the science and art of medicine, on Monday, December 3rd, 1945, by vote of the House of Delegates. I am further directed by the members of the House to convey to you their congratulations, their confidence in your worthiness to receive this award, and their regrets that you were unable to be present in Chicago to accept this medal in a more formal manner and from the hands of the President.

George expressed his gratitude for this new honor, and then he continued:

I do not know how to thank you properly for this dinner. My science began with insects — I should like to tell you a little about butterflies. On November 20 of this year you could have seen me getting out of my car and running across a field on a lovely sunny day. I had seen a butterfly . . . Some time after my collection had been destroyed, Mrs. Minot and I dined with Dr. and Mrs. Edwin J. Cohn and there met Dr. Hisaw [Frederick Lee Hisaw, Professor of Zoology at Harvard], who told me that the insect which destroyed my specimens was a dermestid — a very small beetle known as a "carpet beetle" . . . Tonight I feel as small as a dermestid and as snug as a bug in a rug amidst so many friends . . .

The invitation to this sixtieth-birthday dinner included the request that each person invited write to George a letter, partly to send congratulations but even more to make a statement of what George had meant to him. These letters form a most interesting collection, and at the dinner the package containing them was given to George. The plan was to have the letters bound in a handsome leather volume of quarto size, but unfortunately the book could not be ready in time. After the volume was completed, anyone who called on George could see the immense pleasure that it gave him. Today this volume of letters is one of Mrs. Minot's most cherished possessions.

In February 1946, George talked on the radio again, this time on a program sponsored by the Lederle Laboratories, entitled "The Doctors Talk It Over." It was an excellent question-and-answer conversation, with Mr. Milton Cross asking about blood cells and their origin, as well as about pernicious anemia and its treatment with liver, and with Dr. Minot's intelligent answers. During the next week or two, he was surprised to receive so many letters from patients asking for suggestions about their own symptoms.

His friend, Dr. William T. Salter, at Yale, wrote: "We were delighted and greatly surprised yesterday to hear your well-known voice telling the world about anemia. We were quite interested in your lay presentation. In fact, I think quite a few doctors probably learned something."

Mr. Guy Emerson, of the Bankers' Trust Company, a classmate in the Harvard Class of 1908, wrote: "Dear George: I was delighted to hear you on the radio yesterday. You managed to get over your talk so that it sounded very intimate and human, almost like a personal conversation. It was abundantly clear, even to a layman, and I want to send you a word of congratulation on it."

In reply, George wrote: "Dear Guy: You are a thoughtful fellow. Indeed it is a long time since I have heard from you, although it seems only yesterday that I saw you. I am glad that you appreciate the work in trying to get a manuscript in order and the proper links suitable to the radio audience. I think I spoke a little better than usual over the radio because I have had other persons write to me the nice remarks that you have made."

In April 1946, George had accepted an invitation to talk to the doctors in New Bedford, and he wrote a very characteristic letter to Dr. Russell Wood:

> To be forehanded, I am writing to ask you where I should plan to meet you on May 1st. As I understand it, I am to speak at 5:00 o'clock, and I am assuming I am to speak for about an hour.
>
> I plan to come by motor. I have a new chauffeur coming at the end of this week, so he will be pretty new to me on May 1st. I shall certainly not encourage him to go fast, and so I will allow lots of time coming back from New Bedford. I will expect to take some food with me to eat before I get back to my residence in Brookline, so I feel I should leave New Bedford pretty promptly by shortly after 6:00 o'clock. I remember your mentioning you might be kind enough to ask me to have some dinner in New Bedford, and I simply am letting you know that I think I should start back to Boston as soon as I reasonably can after 6:00 P.M.
>
> I shall plan to show some lantern slides. As I dictate, I am planning to put some lantern slides together over the week end.

The attention to detail is typical. One can be sure that it was written out in order to save Dr. Wood from any possible anxiety about the welfare of his guest. The new chauffeur was Andrew Kelly, a genial Irishman in his thirties who was destined to be of great service to George and Marian.

When the "March of Dimes" for poliomyelitis, the Christmas seals for tuberculosis, the "Jimmy Fund" for cancer in children, as well as the American Heart Association, were all so successful in raising money, it was not long before the champions of other diseases started drives of their own. It was not surprising that in October 1946, George should have a letter requesting his help in organizing a "National Society for the Study of Blood and Its Disorders." The idea did not appeal to him: "I am sorry to say that I would not be interested . . . The only comments I have are that I think it is a mistake to have a series of national organizations for the study of special conditions."

On Wednesday, April 16, 1947, shortly after breakfast, George was sitting quietly reading his paper before starting for the hospital. It was a normal morning; he had enjoyed his breakfast; he felt as well as usual and was not aware of any change in his condition. There was no unusual activity, either physical or mental. He was very surprised, therefore, to find that when he tried to get up he could not control his left leg; he could not make it move. The leg felt all right; it did not tingle; it was not numb; there was no pain of any kind; he simply could not move it. Marian came running, and by that time his left arm felt queer too. It was heavy and weak, and in another few minutes he could not use his arm any more than he could use his leg.

He had no headache, no pains anywhere; there was no nausea; he did not lose consciousness; he was not even dizzy. Dr. Stetson arrived in a few minutes, and he and the faithful Andrew carried the patient to his bed. The paralysis resulting from a thrombosis — a clot causing a stoppage of the blood flow — to the right side of his brain was obvious, and bed rest was essential.

My wife and I went out after office hours and found George talkative and cheerful. He told us all about it, and we were pleased to believe that "all was well for the moment" — except of course that Marian was deeply concerned, although she did not show her anxiety and was efficient and helpful as always.

Everyone knew that this was the beginning of the end. George might have another shock within an hour, but it was more likely that he would regain a good deal of the lost function after a recovery period of several weeks. On the other hand, it might be that his left side would be paralyzed for the rest of his life, and he might live for several years. There was no way to tell what would develop, but in any case the future outlook was not cheerful.

It was dreadful to contemplate what had happened and what might happen. His speech was normal on that first afternoon, but on the next day it was thick and slow. Fortunately, however, it returned to normal promptly. Within two or three weeks his condition was reasonably good again, his mind was clear, and his talk was bright and cheerful once more. He knew very well that he could not go to his office at the hospital for a month or more, but it was some time before he became resigned to the fact that his real work was done. In June 1947, two months after the shock, he was optimistic. Concerning a manuscript overdue, he wrote: "I expect to be perfectly well by autumn, and indeed I hope to be out of doors in the country before more than a few days pass by."

The Minots stayed in Brookline all through the hot summer, he moving about the house and out into the garden in his wheelchair. In September he wrote to a friend: "I have been indulging in a thrombosis of the right side of my brain which, I am pleased to say, did not affect my speech or my mental status: I am convinced that my thinking apparatus is working as it usually does. I am sorry that I cannot contribute much information about the men proposed [for the Society]."

In the fall, he was a good deal better. He was becoming adjusted to his wheelchair existence, he could move the chair by himself, his right arm was strong, and he could pull himself into the automobile and out again, even though the transfer was a slow business.

Andrew proved to be a nurse as well as a chauffeur and general handyman, and he soon learned how to help the doctor up and down stairs and in and out of the wheelchair. He knew what crippling disease was, for, some years before, he had sustained a severe back injury from which he had recovered entirely, thanks to excellent treatment in the hospital and in the rehabilitation clinic. He understood well the need for patience and encouragement at the same time. George soon developed a real confidence in Andrew, and the two would take drives together in the back roads of the countryside, going slowly and stopping whenever George saw a bird or a tree, or perhaps a wildflower, that interested him — and that was often.

George was never able to walk by himself again, but with Marian or Andrew holding on to him, he could get around quite well. His left arm and leg pained him; he would let no one touch his left side, and efforts at rehabilitation were not successful. He was confined to his wheelchair. Even so, he could visit his close friends and have them come to him.

Marian was wonderful with him. She could help him move out of the car and into the wheelchair, and then Andrew could pull him up the steps and into the house. George loved company, and in spite of his disability he was genial and talkative. He was interested, and he was interesting.

His stamp collection was resurrected and gave him much pleasure, all the more so when his son Charlie became interested with him. On week ends, especially, Charlie would help his father sort the stamps contained in boxes and envelopes of every size and color. Correspondence about stamps developed, and the professional stamp dealers began to call on George. At times, if it was a nice day, Andrew would drive him in town and help him into the dealer's store. "I spent more money than I intended this morning, but you should see what I found — the collection of U.S. airmails is pretty good now, if I may say so."

Following the sixtieth-birthday dinner, a group of George's colleagues had conceived the idea of publishing an anniversary volume of scientific papers to be written in his honor. The project was quite different from the personal letters; it was in addition to them. George had written the foreword for the first issue of *Blood — The Journal of Hematology,*[2] published in October 1945, and now the editorial board graciously offered their assistance to his friends. A world-wide committee was formed, and each investigator who had added to the knowledge of blood disease was invited to contribute. The *George R. Minot Symposium on Hematology*[3] was published in 1949; it was an assembly of eighty-four articles.

The foreword by Dean C. Sidney Burwell is a warm appraisal of George's qualities. It says in part:

> First of all, George Minot is George Minot. No one in the world is quite like him. He had been surrounded by tradition all his life . . . An insatiable curiosity and an avidity for understanding drove his mind into new and startling regions of thought . . . That his curiosity is a major motive is attested by his writings . . . The desire to explain something otherwise inexplicable is one of the best motives for research, and its validity is shown not only by his classic discovery, but by his capacity to stimulate curiosity in others and to gather around himself young men who have curiosity similar to his own.[4]

The *Symposium,* or *"Festschrift,"* begins with a reprint of the original paper by Minot and Murphy on the "Treatment of Pernicious Anemia by a Special Diet." And then it goes on with papers that trace the history of hematology. It includes most if not all of the important advances made up to the time of publication. The list of 164 authors represents George's friends and co-workers in hematology, and it is impressive to see how many of the contributors owed their interest and their ability to produce new work to their association with the "Chief."

George was not well when the new volume was handed to him, but I can recall the late afternoon when I found him sitting in his wheelchair before the fire with the book in his lap. It was with obvious pleasure and satisfaction that he showed me the title page and then the long list of contributors. Marian was even more pleased; she could understand and appreciate the efforts that so many had made to show their respect and their love to George.

George wrote "thank-you" letters to every one of the contributors. The telephone was a godsend to him, for each morning he could dictate letters of all kinds to his secretary in the Thorndike, talking sometimes for nearly an hour.

He sent a copy of the *Symposium* to his son Charlie, then eighteen years old and a student at Brooks School. The letter that went with the volume showed how pleased he was with this recognition of his accomplishments. It did not, however, include any word about accomplishments of other kinds, such as the training of several hundred young graduates of the Thorndike, all of whom have done well as investigators and teachers of medicine. The letter did not say that as many as forty-six of George's men had been chosen to be professors of medicine in as many medical schools in this country. The letter does not touch on his ability to select these men in the first place, to pick for his staff men who had ample knowledge of medicine and who at the same time were bright, intelligent gentlemen. As said before in this account, more than one friend has suggested that the success of the Thorndike under Peabody and under Minot depended upon the character quite as much as upon the technical abilities of the young men who were appointed to its staff.

One evening when my wife and I were sitting in his study with George in his wheelchair and Marian on the sofa, he was in a chatty mood and his talk made a kind of summary of his own life. I can recall the gist of the conversation:

"Do you realize what extraordinary changes you and I have seen since we graduated? When I think back to our intern days at the M.G.H. and realize that there was literally no research going on in the place at that time, and when I see what is going on today, the contrast is extraordinary. Think of what research in medicine has accomplished — and I mean clinical research at the bedside quite as much as what I might call scientific or technical research in laboratories or in special institutes. Put it this way. Today we know a good deal about pernicious anemia because we know something about the mechanism that causes it, and because of that knowledge we can treat it easily and successfully. You and I have seen with our own eyes the virtual abolition of many diseases and the control of many others — all because of our understanding of the process which is causing the trouble."

"I have another idea," I said. "Think of the money that has been poured into hospitals and research institutes."

"You are quite right," George went on. "Where it all comes from is well known, of course, but I have to think of the faith and the confidence with which Dr. Edsall and all the other heads of departments in our medical schools first began to ask for money for research — and I have to think of the faith and the hope which those who were glad to give the money must have had, in addition to their great generosity.

"Now, of course, times have changed. Generous people have been shown what their contributions have accomplished, and today they are still responding as best they can to the need for more and still more money. Today, of course, we have a much better idea of what we want and why we want it. Our needs call for apparatus and materials which are far more expensive than the simple equipment you and I had in the early days at the M.G.H. or in Baltimore. And then, just think of the technicians and research assistants of all kinds who use the apparatus to apply the new knowledge — who are so necessary for the work program — but who cost money, too. I like to think that the money is being spent wisely."

Dr. George Packer Berry, Dean of the Harvard Medical School since 1949, tells me that, incredible as it seems, today more than one hundred times as many dollars are spent on research at the School as was spent in 1910. The figure has risen from approximately $21,000 in 1910 to about $2,000,000 in 1953–54. George Minot never saw those figures. I am sure he would be pleased to know that his friends, both in and out of the Harvard Medical School, are trying to establish the George Richards Minot Professorship of Medicine in order to perpetuate the attainments reached when men of high standards can work together in an environment that is both friendly and critical. When the Professorship comes into being, one may be sure that he who sits in its chair will feel the guiding hand and heart, as well as the inquisitive spirit, of George Richards Minot.

Meanwhile, the medical students working in the library can look up from their books and see George's portrait, painted by Mr. Charles Hopkinson, hanging on the wall. The pose is formal and the profile is a trifle austere, but the picture depicts a man who enjoyed freedom of thought, speech, and action; a man whose searching spirit led him to investigate the nature of the phenomena which his inquisitive ear and eye had revealed to him; a man who was honest with himself as with others; whose integrity was of a high order; who was a thorough gentleman.

When Dr. Meikeljohn wrote Marian Minot, after George died, he said that in many ways George had been detached from contemporary American life — that George was a survivor of the great cultural tradition of the nineteenth-century Harvard. It is true that George's background did detach him to some extent. It gave him a natural dignity, and his remarkable achievements added to this a sense of authority, which made everybody admire and respect him.

After George died, the officers of the Section on Experimental Medicine and Therapeutics of the American Medical Association established the George Richards Minot Memorial Lectures, with an honorarium made possible by the contributions of his former students. It was very appropriate that the first lecture, given in 1951, was by his loyal associate, Dr. William B. Castle, who described "The Contributions of George Richards Minot to Experimental Medicine." [5] The second lecture, given in 1952, was by Dr. Cyrus C. Sturgis,[6] and the third in 1953 by Dr. Chester S. Keefer,[7] both brilliant disciples of Dr. Minot. George did not know of this "measure of the reverence that thoughtful men hold for the great man and the great physician" — as the editorial[8] in the *New England Journal of Medicine* expressed it at the time.

On that evening in George's study he asked, "Rack! Did you ever look through an electron microscope? Do you remember all the time that I spent looking at the blood platelets? I saw a platelet not long ago under the electron microscope, and I give you my word it looked as big as a house; and as for details, I could see everything — the contents of the cell as well as the structure of the cell membrane which surrounded it. That machine alone will some day give the key to somebody's important problem.

"What do you know about isotopes? I learned about them, too, not long ago. The chemists are having a fine time labeling certain elements by making them radioactive, and then with a thing called a Geiger counter they find the part that these elements play in complex reactions, and the physiologists can trace and identify labeled elements as they pass through the body. It is all beyond me, of course, but goodness knows it is important stuff. There is an isotope room — they call it the 'hot room' because of the radioactive materials in it — already at the Thorndike, and it is telling us about all sorts of interesting things. The way in which the young men know how to apply the remarkable discoveries in the basic sciences like physics and chemistry to our problems in clinical medicine is positively exciting.

George Minot's mind was still active. He was always the inquisitive physician. During most of the three years following his hemiplegia, he was cheerful, and he was interesting. There were times when he was irritable, for too much company and too much activity and excitement were not good for him. Who wouldn't be irritable under such conditions? Throughout a trying period his wife was a skillful manager. She knew when he needed to be entertained by the guests at a dinner party, and when to accept their invitations. George was not always enthusiastic, but she would say, "Of course you can do it. Andrew will help you into the car, and help you into the house when we get there, and we will have a very pleasant evening." She knew also when he had had enough. "Come on now, it is time for me to put you to bed." And all the time she was still watching his food, giving him injections of insulin every morning and every night, nursing his diabetes. More than one has said that Marian Minot deserves her own special prize.

As President of the American Clinical and Climatological Association in 1933, George ended his address with this sentence: "To teach the art of courageous living is often the chief prescription for the patient with chronic arthritis." If ever a man practiced the art of courageous living, it was George Richards Minot.

To the very end he carried on to the limit of his strength and ability, and then on the morning of Saturday, February 25, 1950, Marian telephoned to us: "George died very quietly at 4:45 this morning."

Appendix

Family Background

Two years before he died, Cousin Jim compiled an account of the "Ancestors and Descendants of George Richards Minot [1758–1802]," and most of what follows comes from that account.

George Minott came from England to America in 1630 and settled in Dorchester, the high land in the south part of the present Boston which overlooks the harbor. He was a member of the Great and General Court when, on September 8, 1636, the vote to create Harvard College was passed.

Minot's Light by the entrance to Boston Harbor is on "Minot's Ledge," so named because a ship belonging to "George Minot who owned T Wharf in 1754" was wrecked there. At least that is how Mr. Edward R. Snow explains it in *Minot's Ledge Light* (Boston: Yankee Publishing Company, 1940), p. 109.

The first George Richards Minot (1758–1802), the future Judge Minot, was graduated A.B. from Harvard in 1778, and studied law in the office of the Honorable Judge Tudor. In 1781 he established an office at 38 Court Street in downtown Boston, his sign hanging from the apple tree outside. He wrote a history of Shays' Rebellion, *The Insurrections in Massachusetts in the Year 1786,* and later the *Continuation of the History of the Province of Massachusetts Bay from the Year 1748.* (This was a continuation from the point where Mr. Thomas Hutchinson's history had ended.) I cherish my copies which George gave me one Christmas. When in 1790 Massachusetts had a state lottery, the tickets were signed by George R. Minot, and my George liked to display his collection of them. Judge Minot died in January 1802, when he was only forty-four years old, probably of tuberculosis.

His only son was William Minot (1783–1873), who married Louisa Davis. He was a lawyer and a very successful trustee. He built a house at 61 Beacon Street, and also he established "Woodbourne," a lovely country place out in Forest Hills, a good seven-mile drive from the foot of Beacon Hill. The trains of the Boston and Providence railroad, starting from the old depot in Park Square where the Hotel Statler stands today, stopped at the Forest Hills station. Mr. Minot could reach his office each morning without too much difficulty.

William and Louisa (Davis) Minot had six children. Their three sons were George Richards (1813–1883), William (1817–1894), and Francis (1821–1899). This second George, grandson of the Judge, attended a school in Jamaica Plain kept by Stephen Minot Weld. He and Francis Minot Weld, brother of the headmaster, were of the same age and became lifelong friends. The twin houses which they built in Bar Harbor have been described in Chapter 1. Mr. Minot and Mr. Weld were related. The "Minot" came into the Weld name because Francis' mother was Hannah Minot, whose father, Jonas Clarke Minot, married Hannah Speakman. Hannah Speakman Minot's sister Mary married the Judge — the first George Richards Minot — and so it appears that Francis Minot Weld and the second George Richards Minot had grandmothers who were sisters.

The second George Richards Minot, my George's grandfather, formed with Nathaniel Hooper the partnership of Minot and Hooper, East India Merchants. They owned ships and continued in business as long as the East India trade was the important commerce of Boston. This grandfather had married Harriet Jackson, daughter of Dr. James Jackson, whom Dr. Oliver Wendell Holmes referred to as the "beloved physician." It was this Dr. James Jackson who had joined with Dr. John Collins Warren in founding the Massachusetts General Hospital in 1821. Dr. Jackson was the second Hersey Professor of Theory and Practice of Physic at the Harvard Medical School, succeeding Dr. Benjamin Waterhouse, the champion of smallpox vaccination. George was proud of his direct descent, through only three generations, from Dr. Jackson.

After their marriage, George and Harriet Minot lived in winter on Pinckney Street, opposite Louisburg Square on Beacon Hill, and in spring and fall at Woodbourne. In midsummer they took their family to Bar Harbor to live beside the Welds in the twin houses in "The Field." In 1883 they built a large house at 245 Marlborough Street in Boston, but unfortunately Mr. Minot died, at the age of seventy, just before it was ready. The family, however, moved in shortly afterwards. George and Harriet Minot had eight children, three sons and five daughters. Their seventh child and second son was James Jackson Minot, George's father and my Cousin Jim.

George's great-grandfather William Minot's second son was another William (1817–1894), who married Katherine Maria Sedgwick, a talented woman, author of *Hope Leslie* and other novels about life in New England. More than once I have heard my mother speak of the good times at Woodbourne with her "Uncle William" and "Aunt Kitty." William and Katherine also had seven children. Their second son was Dr. Charles Sedgwick Minot, who became the distinguished embryologist, known throughout the world for his lucid descriptions of the evolution of the various tissues and organs of our body. He was one of the first professors to work in the Harvard Medical School on a full-time basis, and he lectured to our class in the first year there. Out of school he was "Cousin Charles" to both George and me.

William's third son was Dr. Francis Minot (1821–1899). He was a delightful gentleman, with a keen sense of humor, and an excellent practitioner of medicine in Boston. For twenty-nine years he was Visiting Physician to the Massachusetts General Hospital. He was the third Hersey Professor of the Theory and Practice of Physic in the Harvard Medical School, and he was the fourth President of the Association of American Physicians. He married Sarah Parkman Blake, and their only child, Julia, was my mother. George's father and my mother were children of brothers, and George and I were the grandsons of brothers. The Minot family tree, which shows these relationships, is attached.

George Minot's mother was the daughter of Henry Austin Whitney (1826–1889), whose wife was Fanny Lawrence (1828–1883). He was Secretary of the Harvard Class of 1846, and he, too, was a successful businessman. George was always gratified to know that his Grandfather Whitney had been a Trustee of the Massachusetts General Hospital. Both sides of his family, therefore, had been interested in the development of good medical practice in the community. When Mr. Whitney's daughter Elizabeth was married to Dr. James Jackson Minot in 1884, Mr. Whitney built for her the house at 188 Marlborough Street, where George and his brothers were born and lived.

From his forebears George Minot inherited his spirit of inquisitiveness and his industry — his capacity for taking pains; but better than that, he inherited a culture that gave him a sound integrity, a devotion to duty, and a desire to know the truth. The fact that his family had been successful in business and were well-to-do made his material life easy and comfortable. It gave him opportunities not available to all, and he accepted the obligations that went with them. His services to his fellow men were immeasurable.

Minot Genealogy

GEORGE RICHARDS MINOT (The Judge) 1758–1802 m. Mary Speakman 1754–1811

William Minot 1783–1873 m. Louisa Davis 1788–1858

I. Mary 1811–1882

II. GEORGE RICHARDS 1813–1883 m. Harriet Jackson 1813–1886

1. Louisa 1841–1932
2. Hariet 1843–1925
3. Sarah 1845–1903
4. Mary 1846–1919
5. George Richards 1849–1894 m. Agnes Olney 1861–1943
   - Francis 1891–
6. Elizabeth Cabot 1851–1926
7. JAMES JACKSON 1852–1938 m. Elizabeth Whitney 1860–1903
   - GEORGE RICHARDS 1885–1950
   - James Jackson 1891–
   - Henry Whitney 1896–
8. Francis 1854–1884

III. William 1817–1894 m. Katherine Maria Sedgwick 1820–1880

1. Jane 1844–1847
2. Alice 1847–1883
3. William 1849–1900 m. Elizabeth V. VanPelt 1858–1897
   - Katherine 1883–
   - William 1885–1937
   - Vrendenburgh 1887–1928
   - Sedgwick 1891–
4. CHARLES S. 1852–1914 m. Lucy Fosdick 1858–1939
5. Robert S. 1856–1910 m. Abbey H. Manning 1861–1942
   - Robert S. 1886–
   - Wayland M. 1889–
   - Henry Davis 1890–1953
   - Ruth 1892–1892
6. Henry Davis 1859–1890
7. Lawrence 1865–1921

IV. Francis 1818–1819

V. Francis 1821–1899 m. Sarah Parkman Blake 1833–1869

1. Julia 1863–1945 m. Felix Rackemann 1861–1934
   - Francis M. 1887–
   - Elizabeth 1890–1897
   - Sarah P. 1892–

VI. Julia 1823–1875

References

Chapter 1. In the Beginning

1. Minot, G. R., "The Chrysalis of Melitaea Gabbi," *Entomological News 13,* 158 (May 1902).
2. Minot, G. R., "The Tussock Moth Peril," Letter to the Editor, *Boston Evening Transcript* (Feb. 21, 1903).

Chapter 3. Harvard Medical School

1. Cannon, Walter B., *The Wisdom of the Body* (New York: Norton, 1932). Contains references to his important papers.
2. Henderson, Lawrence J., *Blood: a Study in General Physiology* (New Haven: Yale University Press, 1928).
3. Folin, Otto, *Laboratory Manual of Biological Chemistry* (New York: Appleton, ed. 5, 1934).
4. Osler, William, *The Principles and Practice of Medicine* (New York: Appleton, ed. 1, 1892). There were many editions. We studied the seventh, of 1909.
5. Frothingham, C., Jr., and Minot, G. R., "Normal Temperature of Rabbits," *Am. J. Physiol. 30,* 430 (1912).
6. Frothingham, C., Jr., and Minot, G. R., "The Effect of the Injection of Bovine Bile into Rabbits," *J. Med. Research 22,* 79 (1912).
7. Smith, Theobald, and Kilborne, F. L., *Investigations into the Nature, Causation and Prevention of Texas or Southern Cattle Fever* (Washington: U. S. Department of Agriculture Bulletin No. 1, Government Printing Office, 1893).
8. Cabot, R. C., *Case Teaching in Medicine* (Boston: Heath, 1908), pp. vii–ix.
9. Wright, J. H., "Origin and Nature of the Blood Platelets," *Boston M. & S. J. 154,* 643 (1906).

Chapter 4. Massachusetts General Hospital

1. Garland, J. E., "The Story of a Hospital," *Harvard Alumni Bull. 48,* 3 (1946).
2. Massachusetts General Hospital case records analyzed by the author.
3. Means, J. H., *The Thyroid and Its Diseases* (Philadelphia: Lippincott, 1937), p. 139.

REFERENCES

Chapter 5. Baltimore

1. Lee, R. I., and White, P. D., "A Clinical Study of the Coagulation Time of the Blood," *Am. J. Med. Sci. 145,* 495 (1913).
2. Fitz, R., in Washburn, F. A., *The Massachusetts General Hospital, Its Development 1900–1935* (Boston: Houghton Mifflin, 1939), p. 185.
3. Newburgh, L. H., and Minot, G. R., "The Blood Pressure in Pneumonia," *Arch. Int. Med. 14,* 48 (1914).
4. Snowden, R. Personal letter.
5. Minot, G. R., "Nitrogen Metabolism Before and After Splenectomy in a Case of Pernicious Anemia," *Bull. Johns Hopkins Hosp. 25,* 285 (1914).
6. Denny, G. P., and Minot, G. R., "The Origin of Antithrombin," *Am. J. Physiol. 38,* 233 (1915).
7. Minot, G. R., and Rackemann, F. M., "Respiratory Signs and Symptoms in Trichinosis," *Am. J. Med. Sci. 150,* 571 (1915).

Chapter 6. Research at M.G.H. and Huntington

1. Flexner, Abraham, *Medical Education in the United States and Canada. A Report to the Carnegie Foundation for the Advancement of Teaching* (New York: Carnegie Foundation for the Advancement of Teaching, Bull. No. 4, 1910).
2. Rogers, O., Personal letter.
3. Kerr, W. J., Personal letter.
4. Minot, G. R., "Methods of Testing Donors for Transfusions of Blood and Consideration of Factors Influencing Agglutinations and Hemolysis," *Boston M. & S. J. 174,* 667 (1916).
5. Minot, G. R., "Studies on a Case of Idiopathic Purpura Hemorrhagica," *Am. J. Med. Sci. 152,* 48 (1916).
6. Lee, R. I., Minot, G. R., and Beth Vincent, "Splenectomy in Pernicious Anemia. Studies on Bone Marrow Stimulation," *J.A.M.A. 67,* 719 (1916).
7. Lee, R. I., and Minot, G. R., "The Blood Platelets in Hemophilia," *Arch. Int. Med. 18,* 474 (1916).
8. Castle, W. B., "The Contribution of George Richards Minot to Experimental Medicine," New England *J. Med. 247,* 585 (1952).
9. Minot, G. R., "Diminished Blood Platelets and Marrow Insufficiency. A Classification and Differential Diagnosis of Purpura Hemorrhagica, Aplastic Anemia, and Allied Conditions," *Arch. Int. Med. 19,* 1062 (1917).
10. Wright, J. H., and Minot, G. R., "The Viscous Metamorphosis of the Blood Platelets," *J. Exper. Med. 36,* 395 (1917).
11. Hamilton, Alice, *Industrial Poisons in the United States* (New York: Macmillan, 1925).
12. Minot, G. R., "Blood Examinations of Trinitrotoluene Workers," *J. Indust. Hyg. 1,* 301 (1919).
13. Hamilton, Alice, and Minot, G. R., "Ether Poisoning in the Manufacture of Smokeless Powder," *J. Indust. Hyg. 2,* 41 (1920).

14. Minot, G. R., and Loeb, R. F., "An Attempt to Prevent Influenza at Harvard College," *Boston M. & S. J. 179,* 665 (1918).
15. Peabody, F. W., "The Care of the Patient," *J.A.M.A. 88,* 877 (1927).
16. Collis P. Huntington Memorial Hospital, First Annual Report (1912).

Chapter 7. Diabetes

1. Joslin, E. P., Root, H. F., White, P., and Marble, A., *The Treatment of Diabetes Mellitus* (Philadelphia: Lea & Febiger, ed. 9, 1952).
2. Allen, F. M., *Glycosuria and Diabetes* (Boston: W. M. Leonard, 1913).
3. Banting, F. G., Best, C. H., Collip, J. B., Campbell, W. R., Fletcher, A. A., MacLeod, J. J. R., and Nobel, E. C. "The Effect Produced on Diabetes by Extracts of Pancreas," *Tr. A. Am. Physicians 37,* 337 (1922).
4. Barron, Moses, "The Relation of the Islets of Langerhans to Diabetes with Special Reference to Cases of Pancreatic Lithiasis," *Surg. Gynec. and Obst. 31,* 437 (1920).
5. Pratt, J. H., Unpublished paper.
6. Joslin, E. P., *The Treatment of Diabetes Mellitus* (Philadelphia: Lea & Febiger, ed. 1, 1916), chap. 2
7. Minot, G. R., "Clinical Discussion of the Anemias," *The Oxford Medicine* (New York: Oxford University Press, 1920), vol. 11, pp. 589–679.
8. Minot, G. R., and Lee, R. I. in *The Nelson Loose-Leaf Living Medicine* (New York: Nelson 1920 et seq.).
9. Minot, G. R., and Bock, A. V., "Transfusion of Blood," in Barker, L. F., Hoskins, R. G., and Mosenthal, H. O., eds., *Endocrinology and Metabolism* (New York: Appleton, 1922), vol. 3, p. 821
10. These notes taken from George's files.
11. Minot, G. R., Buckman, T. E., and Isaacs, R., "Chronic Myelogenous Leukemia: Age Incidence, Duration, and Benefit Derived from Irradiation," *J.A.M.A. 82,* 1489–1494 (1924).
12. Minot, G. R., and Isaacs, R., "Lymphatic Leukemia: Age Incidence, Duration and Benefit Derived from Irradiation," *Boston M. & S. J. 191,* 1–9 (1924).
13. Minot, G. R., and Isaacs, R., "Lymphoblastoma (Malignant Lymphoma): Age and Sex Incidence, Duration of Disease, and Effect of Roentgenray and Radium Irradiation and Surgery," *J.A.M.A. 82,* 1489–1494 (1924).
14. von Mering and Minkowski, "Diabetes Mellitus nach Pankreasextirpation," *Arch. f. exp. Path. u. Pharmakol. 26,* 371 (1889–90).
15. Collis P. Huntington Memorial Hospital, Thirteenth Annual Report (1925).

Chapter 8. Pernicious Anemia

1. Castle, W. B., "The Contributions of George Richards Minot to Experimental Medicine," *New England J. Med. 247,* 585 (1952).
2. Minot, G. R., and Murphy, W. P., "Treatment of Pernicious Anemia by a Special Diet," *J.A.M.A. 87,* 470 (1926).

3. Hunter, F. T., in Washburn, F. A., *The Massachusetts General Hospital: Its Development 1900–1935* (Boston: Houghton Mifflin, 1939), p. 192.
4. Murphy, W. P., and Minot, G. R. "A Special Diet for Patients with Pernicious Anemia," *Boston M. & S. J. 195,* 410 (1926).
5. Minot, G. R., and Murphy, W. P., "A Diet Rich in Liver in the Treatment of Pernicious Anemia — Study of One Hundred and Five Cases," *J.A.M.A. 89,* 759 (1927).
6. Fenwick, Samuel, "Atrophy of the Stomach," *Lancet 2,* 78 (1870).
7. Fenwick, Samuel, *Atrophy of the Stomach and on the Nervous Affection of the Digestive Organs* (London: Churchill, 1880).
8. Gibson, R. B., and Howard, C. P., "Metabolic Studies in Pernicious Anemia," *Arch. Int. Med. 32,* 1 (1923).
9. Stockman, R., "Observations on the Causes and Treatment of Chlorosis," *Brit. M. J. 2,* 1473 (1895).
10. Millspaugh, C. F., *Medicinal Plants: An Illustrated and Descriptive Guide to Plants Indigenous to and Naturalized in the United States which are Used in Medicine* (Philadelphia: John C. Yorston & Co., 1892).

Chapter 9. The Thorndike Memorial Laboratory

1. Peabody, F. W., Clough, H. D., Sturgis, C. C., Wearn, J. T., and Tompkins, E. H., "Effect of Epinephrine on Soldiers with Irritable Heart," *J.A.M.A. 71,* 1912, 1918). (Note that Peabody was observing soldiers rather than hearts!)
2. Peabody, F. W., "The Function of a Municipal Hospital," *Boston M. & S. J. 189,* 125 (1923).
3. Peabody, F. W., "The Care of the Patient," *J.A.M.A. 88,* 877 (1927; Cambridge: Harvard University Press, 1927).
4. *A Memoir, Francis Weld Peabody 1881–1927* (Privately printed at the Riverside Press, Cambridge, 1933).
5. Peabody, F. W., "The Soul of the Clinic," *J.A.M.A. 90,* 1193 (1928).
6. Blumgart, H. L., and Weiss, S., "Studies on the Velocity of Blood Flow," *J. Clin. Invest.* (1927); several papers.
7. Ferris, E. B., Jr., Capps, R. B., and Weiss, S. "Carotid Sinus Syncope and Its Bearing on the Mechanism of the Unconscious State and Convulsions," *Medicine 14,* 377 (1935).
8. Wearn, J. T., "The Extent of the Capillary Bed of the Heart," *J. Exper. Med. 47,* 273 (1928).
9. Minot, G. R., *The Treatment of Pernicious Anemia.* The Harvey Society Publications (New York) *23,* 151 (1929).
10. Minot, G. R., "Remarks upon Acceptance of the Kober Medal," *Tr. A. Am. Physicians 44,* 11 (1929).
11. Mettier, S. R., Minot, G. R., and Townsend, W. C. "Scurvy in Adults, Especially the Effect of Food Rich in Vitamin C on Blood Formation," *J.A.M.A. 95,* 1089 (1930).
12. Minot, G. R., and Heath, C. W., "The Response of the Reticulocytes to Iron," *Am. J. M. Sc. 133,* 110 (1932).

13. Jackson, James, "On a Peculiar Disease Resulting from the Use of Ardent Spirits," *New England J. Med. and Surg.* (1822).
14. Strauss, M. B., and McDonald, W. J., "Polyneuritis of Pregnancy, A Dietary Deficiency Disorder," *J.A.M.A. 100,* 1320 (1933).
15. Minot, G. R., Strauss, M. B., and Cobb, S., "'Alcoholic' Polyneuritis: Dietary Deficiency as a Factor in its Production," *New England J. Med. 208,* 1244 (1933).
16. Strauss, M. B., "The Etiology of 'Alcoholic' Polyneuritis," *J. Clin. Investigation 13,* 696 (1934).
17. Benson, E. F., *Queen Victoria's Daughters* (New York: Appleton-Century-Crofts, 1938).
18. Rosenthal, R. L., "Hemophilia and Hemophilia-like Diseases Caused by Deficiencies in Plasma Thromboplastic Factors: Antihemophilic Globulin (AHG), Antecedent (PTA)," *Am. J. Med. 17,* 57 (1954).
19. Lee, R. I., and Minot, G. R., "The Blood Platelets in Hemophilia," *Arch. Int. Med. 18,* 474 (1916).
20. Patek, A. J., Jr., and Stetson, R. P., "Hemophilia I. The Abnormal Coagulation of the Blood and Its Relation to the Blood Platelets," *J. Clin. Investigation 15,* 531 (1936).
21. Patek, A. J., Jr., and Taylor, F. H. L., "Hemophilia II. Some Properties of a Substance Obtained from Normal Human Plasma Effective in Accelerating the Coagulation of Hemophilic Blood," *J. Clin. Investigation 16,* 113 (1937).
22. Cecil, R. L., ed., *Text-Book of Medicine* (Philadelphia: Saunders, eds. 1–7, 1927–1947).
23. Minot, G. R. in Cecil's Medicine (ed. 7, 1947), p. 1100.
24. Harrington, W. J., Minnich, V., Hollingsworth, J. W., and Moore, C. V., "Demonstrations of a Thrombocytopenic Factor in the Blood of Patients with Idiopathic Thrombocytopenic Purpura," *J. Lab. & Clin. Med. 36,* 1 (1951).

Chapter 10. Extracurricular Busyness

1. Cohn, Edwin J., *et al.,* "The Nature of the Material Effective in Pernicious Anemia," *Abstracts of the Communications of the 13th International Physiological Congress* (Boston, August 19–24, 1929), p. 55.
2. "Sesquicentenary of the Professorship of the Theory and Practice of Physic," *Harvard Medical Alumni Bulletin 7,* 17 (January 1933).
3. Jackson, James, *Letters to a Young Physician* (Boston: Phillips, Sampson & Co., 1855).
4. Minot, G. R., "The Importance of Art and the General Principles of Treatment in Chronic Arthritis," President's Address, *Tr. Am. Clin. and Climat. A. 49,* 50 (1933).
5. Minot, G. R., "Anemias of Nutritional Deficiency," Gordon Wilson Lecture, *Tr. Am. Clin. and Climat. A. 55,* 175 (1940).
6. Minot, G. R., Address in *The Celebration of the Dedication of the New Lilly Research Laboratories* (Indianapolis: Privately printed, 1934).
7. De Kruif, P., *Men Against Death* (New York: Harcourt, Brace, 1932), pp. 88–116.

REFERENCES

Chapter 11. Nobel Prize

1. *Boston Sunday Advertiser,* October 28, 1934.
2. Minot, G. R., "Discours" Le Banquet Nobel en 1934, *Les Prix Nobel en 1934* (Stockholm: Imprimerie Royale, 1935), p. 58.
3. Minot, G. R., "The Development of Liver Therapy in Pernicious Anaemia — A Nobel Lecture," *Les Prix Nobel en 1934* (Stockholm: Imprimerie Royale, 1935), p. 1; reprinted in *Lancet 1,* 361 (1935).

Chapter 12. The Professor — In Full Stride

1. Cecil, R. L., ed., *Text-Book of Medicine* (Philadelphia: Saunders, ed. 1, 1927; ed. 7, 1947).
2. Minot, G. R., "Clinical Investigation: Physician and Patient. The Ninth Alpha Omega Alpha Annual Lecture," *J.A.M.A. 105,* 641 (1935).
3. Minot, G. R., "The President's Address," *Tr. A. Am. Physicians 53,* 1 (1938).
4. Berry, G. P., "Financing the Harvard Medical School," *Harvard Medical Alumni Bulletin 29,* 7 (1955).
5. Minot, G. R., "Problems of Nutritional Deficiencies," *Publ. A. Nerv. and Ment. Dis. 22,* 29 (1943).
6. These letters from Dr. Vaughan and Dr. Meikeljohn were published subsequently in the *Lancet* for March 4 and March 11, 1950, respectively.
7. Personal letter to the author.

Chapter 13. Recognition of Authority

1. A transcript of the proceedings was incorporated with the letters of greeting which Dr. Castle collected for Dr. Minot.
2. Minot, G. R., "Foreword," *Blood — The Journal of Hematology 1,* 1 (1946).
3. Dameshek, W., and Taylor, F. H. L., eds., *George R. Minot Symposium on Hematology* (New York: Grune & Stratton, 1949).
4. Burwell, C. Sidney, "Foreword," *George R. Minot Symposium on Hematology;* reprinted in *Blood — The Journal of Hematology 3,* 5 (1949).
5. Castle, W. B., "The Contributions of George Richards Minot to Experimental Medicine," Presented as the first George R. Minot Lecture of the Section on Experimental Medicine and Therapeutics at the Annual Meeting of the American Medical Association, Atlantic City, New Jersey, June 14, 1951, *New England J. Med. 247,* 585 (1952).
6. Sturgis, C. C., "Some Aspects of the Leukemia Problem," The Second George R. Minot Lecture, *J.A.M.A. 150,* 1551 (1952).
7. Keefer, C. S., "Present Day Treatment of Subacute Bacterial Endocarditis," The Third George R. Minot Lecture, *J.A.M.A. 152,* 1397 (1953).
8. Editorial, "George R. Minot Lectureship," *New England J. Med. 247,* 621 (1952).
9. Minot, G. R., "President's Address: The Importance of Art and the General Principles of Treatment in Chronic Arthritis," *Tr. Am. Clin. and Clim. A. 49,* 1 (1933).

Index

INDEX

INDEX

INDEX

INDEX

INDEX